RENAL DIET COOKBOOK

Improve the Kidney Function to Avoid Dialysis is Possible. 215+ Healthy Recipes & 30-Day Meal Plan to Repair the Kidneys Naturally. Includes a Special Section for Vegan & Vegetarian

BY MICHELLE BURNS

Table of Contents

INTRODUCTION

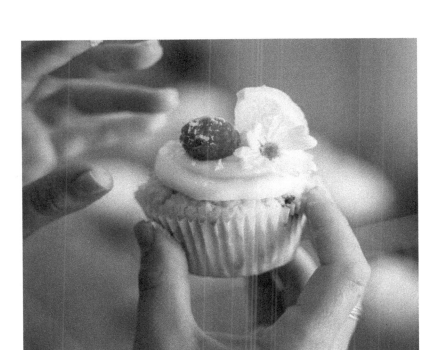

The main principle of the renal diet is to replace canned and processed foods with fresh or frozen fruits and vegetables.

Besides, the renal diet might even be called the most cutting-edge healthy diet because it doesn't allow eating processed food.

Note that this diet limits the use of certain products, but the list of them is rather short. So you will enjoy your life without any solid limitations regarding food and drinks.

Kidney failure has no treatment to reverse it, and it is essential to take a truly healthy diet that protects your body from any kind of health hazards associated with kidney disease. However, if you suffer from kidney failure or any other kidney disease, there is no reason to give up hope; with proper treatment and diet, you can manage it and live a healthy and long life.

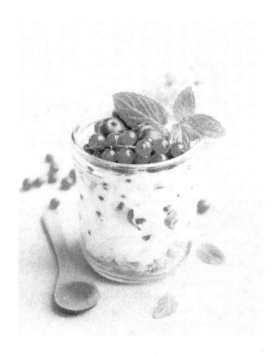

All you have to do is start making healthy lifestyle choices, and it begins with healthy changes to your diet. The good news is that once you start your kidney treatment and maintain your ideal diet, its associated symptoms start to go away.

Good dietary habits are known to keep kidney diseases at bay. It's time to make smart choices when it comes to food that you eat every day. An ideal renal diet is all about including wholesome foods and reducing the number of products which contain high sodium, high phosphorus or high potassium.

An ideal renal diet restricts foods that are harmful to your kidneys and renal system. This exclusive book on renal diet is based on recipes that reduce the consumption of sodium, phosphorus and potassium, and provide your body with healthy nutrients to avoid unwanted health symptoms and complications.

Explore the collection of healthy, homemade recipes for chronic kidney diseases. The purpose of these recipes is to avoid stress to your kidneys without compromising on taste value.

This book provides a comprehensive list of kidney-friendly foods to buy. The recipes are simple to cook and contain everyday ingredients; you don't need to buy exotic, expensive products to consume a healthy renal diet. The recipes will help you maintain the right balance of nutrients so that your kidneys can function efficiently.

Feast your eyes on delicious recipes and enjoy a healthy renal diet.

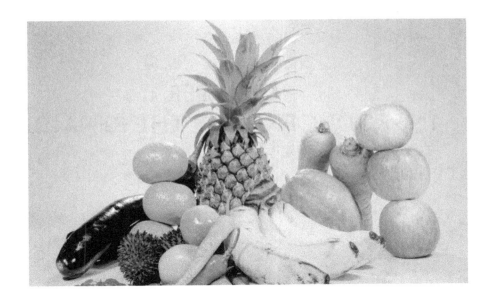

In this book, you will find a meal plan and easy recipes for each day of the month. Even with kidney problems, you can eat delicious food.

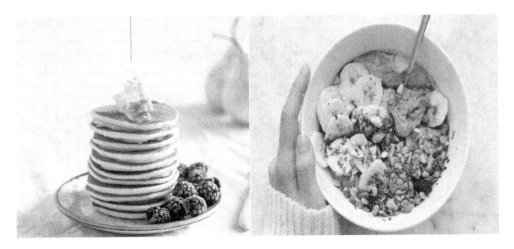

The renal diet is a popular diet plan that can be used as an alternative treatment for different kidney diseases. This is basically a low-sodium, low-potassium, low-phosphorus and low-protein diet that is recommended for people with end-stage kidney diseases. The kidney diet also encourages people to consume high-quality protein and limit fluid and fat intake. The kidney-friendly diet can be restrictive; however, the rewards are oftentimes commendable.

All the information presented in this book is well- researched and based on existing facts and figures in the modern world.

CHAPTER 1:
INTRODUCTION TO THE RENAL DIET

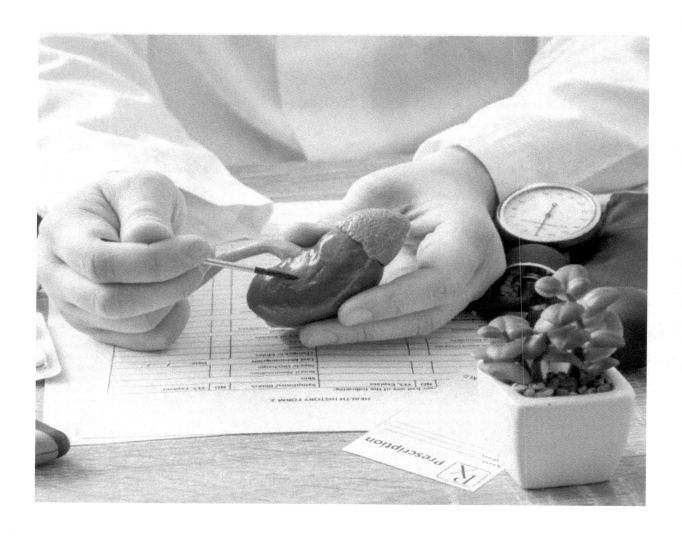

THE RENAL DIET

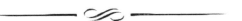

The Renal Diet, also referred to as Kidney Diet or Kidney-Friendly Diet, is a type of diet that restricts a person's intake of sodium, potassium, Phosphorus and protein. This diet lifestyle also focuses on the importance of consuming high-quality protein and limiting fluids. The kidney diet is specifically designed for people with compromised kidney function, specifically those with chronic kidney failure and end-stage kidney disease. The said diet aims to reduce the buildup of micronutrient wastes in the blood to prevent complications like hypertension, fluid overload, irregular heart rhythm, bone diseases and vascular calcification.

A renal diet is an eating plan exercised to help minimize waste products' levels in the blood.

The renal diet is designed to cause as little work or stress on the kidneys as possible, while still providing energy and the high nutrients the body needs.

A renal diet follows several fundamental guidelines. The first is that it must be a balanced, healthy and sustainable diet, rich in natural grains, vitamins, fibers, carbohydrates, omega 3 fats and fluids. Proteins should be adequate, but not excessive.

Accumulates in the blood are kept to a minimum. Blood electrolyte levels are monitored regularly and the diet corrected. It is essential to follow specific advice from your doctor and dietitian.

Daily protein intake is essential to rebuild tissues but needs to be kept to a minimum. Superfluous proteins need to be broken down by the body into nitrates and carbohydrates. Nitrates are not employed by the body and have to be excreted via the kidneys.

Carbohydrates are an important source of energy and should be taken in adequate amounts. Whole grains are the best. Avoid highly refined carbohydrates.

Table salt ought to be limited to cooking only. Excess salt overworks the kidneys and causes fluid retention. Salty foods, like processed meats, sausages and snacks should be avoided.

Phosphorus is essential for the body to function, but dialysis can't remove it, so its amounts need to be monitored, and intake should be restricted though not eliminated completely.

Foods like dairy products, darker drinks such as colas and legumes have high phosphorus content. If levels of this increase in the blood, foods high in potassium, such as citrus fruits and dark, leafy green lettuce, carrots or apricots might have to be restricted.

Omega 3 fats are a significant part of any healthy diet. Fish is an excellent source. Omega fats are important for the body. Avoid trans-fats or hydrolyzed fats.

Fluids should be taken regularly, but might need to be limited in cases of fluid retention.

A healthy renal diet can help keep kidney function for longer. The main differences between a renal diet and any nutritious diet plan are the limitations placed on protein and table salt ingestion. Restrictions on fluids and potassium might become necessary as signs and symptoms of accumulation become evident.

For people with diabetes who also suffer from kidney disease, there is a food strategy or diet. Over fifty percent of chronic kidney disease sufferers are people that have diabetes, indicating the necessity for them to stick to the diabetic diet.

In several cases, this diet is prepared and is effective in different phases of this disease. There are also instances where the diet is created for diabetics hoping to avoid renal disorder. Sufferers from diabetes and kidney problems have trouble eating proper food.

The aim of a diabetic's meal plan would be to get the blood within the safe selection. This may be carried out just by having meals frequently on a daily basis, not missing any, and eating carbohydrate foods that are low glycemic.

Consuming a number of such carbohydrates at every meal can assist the body in maintaining a moderate blood sugar level, becoming neither too high nor too low.

Low glycemic foods include brown rice, sweet potatoes and whole-grain bread. But if it is a renal diet for diabetics, whole-grain bread and sweet potatoes ought not to be used since they're rich in potassium.

People with kidney issues should eat less of these foods full of potassium, phosphorus and sodium. A blood-sugar-lowering diet for people with diabetes can be a diet suitable for renal issues. Patients need to check the labels since sodium is common in many foods.

For clients with kidney problems, dietitians advise against the consumption of diet pops of java because such drinks contain sodium.

On a diabetic-renal meal plan, unsweetened teas, water and diet sodas are allowed. When it comes to vegetables, broccoli, cauliflower, beets, eggplant and cabbage are usually recommended because of their abundant vitamin content and very low carbohydrate and potassium content. Meats that are rich in sodium, such as organ meats, sausage and bacon, ought not to be taken.

Since canned vegetables contain lots of sodium, it is necessary to choose raw vegetables and steer clear of the canned variety. Furthermore, raw vegetables are more nutritious, considering their vitamins.

It is recommended that diabetics learn from certified nutritionists the foods that they need to eat or avoid.

However, all forms of renal diet have one thing in common, which is to improve your renal functions, bring some relief to your kidneys, as well as prevent kidney disease in patients with numerous risk factors, thus improving your overall health and wellbeing. The grocery list we have provided should help you get a hold of which groceries you should introduce to your diet and which groups of food should be avoided in order to improve your kidneys' performance, so you can start shopping for your new lifestyle.

You don't need to shop many different types of groceries all at once as it is always better to use fresh produce, although frozen food also makes a good alternative when fresh fruit and vegetables are not available.

As for the renal diet we are recommending in our guide, this form of kidney-friendly dietary regimen offers solutions in the form of low-sodium and low-potassium meals and groceries, which is why we are also offering simple and easy renal diet recipes in our guide. Follow a dietary plan compiled for all stages of renal system failure, unless your doctor recommends a different treatment by allowing or expelling some of the groceries we have listed in our ultimate grocery list for renal patients.

Before we get to cooking and changing your lifestyle from the very core, with the idea of improving your health, we want you to get familiar with renal diet basics and find out exactly what this diet is based on, while you already know what the very core solution found in renal diet helping you improve your kidney's health by lowering sodium and potassium intake is.

People with impaired kidney function should strictly follow a renal diet to reduce wastes in their blood. These wastes mostly come from the foods and liquids they consume. When your kidneys don't work properly, they are unable to filter the wastes from the foods you eat. These wastes will remain in the blood and will just circulate in your body. If left untreated, this will result in severe complications and can be fatal. The renal diet helps people with kidney problems maintain normal levels of sodium, potassium and proteins in their blood and limit their protein and fluid intake.

Following a kidney-friendly diet also helps reduce the number of dialysis sessions (per week) of those with end-stage kidney disease.

RENAL DIET BASICS

People with kidney problems need to limit or monitor their intake of the following nutrients:

ORANGE & ALMOND COBBLER

Sodium is an important element needed by all living organisms to regulate the water flow in the body. This essential mineral is mostly found in natural foods like salt, but it is present in almost all kinds of food. Processed foods like ham, sausage and bacon contain higher levels of sodium because of their high salt content. Sodium is one of the three major electrolytes of the body, together with potassium and chloride. It helps regulate blood pressure, blood volume, nerve and muscle function and the acid-base balance of the blood. Experts recommend limiting one's intake of sodium to less than (<) 2, 000 mg/day.

Too much sodium can be extremely detrimental for people with kidney problems because this can cause fluid retention in the body. This can further lead to swelling, cardiac overload, high blood pressure and respiratory failure. To monitor your sodium intake, you must do the following: Make sure to check the food labels. Sodium content is always included in the list.

Consume only small servings of different food recipes and know their sodium content.

Avoid consuming canned goods and processed foods because they contain high amounts of sodium.

Choose fresh plant foods, fresh fruits, vegetables, nuts, etc.

Cook or prepare your food at home and do not add salt. Use spices instead. Limit your sodium intake to 350 mg/meal.

POTASSIUM

Potassium is a mineral that helps maintain a regular heartbeat and good muscular function. This element also plays an essential role in maintaining fluid-electrolyte balance in the bloodstream. The kidneys naturally regulate the levels of potassium in your body and expel the excess amounts into the urine. When your kidneys are not working well, they cannot remove excess potassium from your body. This can result in hyperkalemia or high potassium levels in the blood. High levels of potassium can lead to muscle weakness, slow pulse and irregular heart rhythm. If not managed immediately, this can lead to cardiac arrest and death. It is recommended to limit a person's potassium intake to less than (<) 2000 mg/day.

Patients who have kidney problems, especially those with end-stage renal disease should monitor their potassium levels regularly. Here are some tips to keep your potassium levels in the blood safe or within normal range:

Limit foods that contain high amounts of potassium such as bananas, avocados, milk and dairy products.

Do not use salt substitutes and seasonings containing potassium.

Check the potassium or potassium chloride content on different food labels. Eat smaller servings of foods.

Consult your renal dietitian regularly and have your potassium levels checked.

FATS

When you are going through times where you have to restrict what you eat, it is good to know that healthy fats are another macronutrient that you need to include daily. Eating healthy fats makes sure you are getting all the essential fatty acids that can help your body in many ways. Polyunsaturated and monounsaturated fats are both unsaturated fats, but they are healthy fats because of their benefits to the heart like decreasing LDL, increasing HDL and lowering the total cholesterol levels. The correct types of fat might decrease inflammation within the body and will protect your kidneys from more damage. You should try to include small amounts of these fats into your daily diet.

CAR BOH YDRATES

Carbs are another macronutrient that the body needs. This is what the body uses for energy. They also give the body many minerals, fiber, and vitamins that help protect it. The body needs 130 grams of carbs daily for normal function.

SUPPLEMENTS AND VITAMINS

Instead of relying on supplements, you need to follow a balanced diet. This is the best way to get the amount of vitamins your body needs each day. Because of the restrictive CKD diet, it can be hard to get the necessary nutrients and vitamins you need. Anyone who has CKD will have greater needs for vitamins that are water- soluble. Certain renal supplements are needed to get the needed extra water-soluble vitamins. Renal vitamins could be small doses of vitamin C, biotin, pantothenic acid, niacin, folic acid, Vitamins B12, B6, B2 and B1.

Kidneys normally convert inactive vitamin D to an active vitamin D so our bodies can use it. With CKD, kidneys lose the ability to do this. Your health care provider could check your parathyroid hormone, phosphorus and calcium levels to figure out if you need to take any supplements of active vitamin D. This type of vitamin D requires a prescription.

If your doctor hasn't prescribed a supplement, don't hesitate to ask them if you would benefit from one. To help keep you healthy, only use supplements that have been approved by your dietitian or doctor.

PHOSPHORUS

Phosphorus is a mineral that helps maintain bone health and development. It works together with calcium and Vitamin D to keep your bones healthy and strong. It also aids in muscle movement and assists in the formation of connective tissues and organs in the body. Patients with kidney problems typically have elevated phosphorus levels in their blood. When kidneys are compromised, they cannot expel the excess phosphorus out of your body. Too much phosphorus in the blood can result in weak and brittle bones. This can also lead to abnormal calcium deposits in the blood vessels, eyes, heart and lungs. If not properly managed, this can be fatal. The recommended dietary phosphorus intake for a person is between 800-1,000 mg/ day.

Here are the tips to keep your phosphorus at safe, normal levels.

Limit the consumption of foods that are high in phosphorus, such as meat, milk, cheese and canned fish.

Consume smaller servings of high-protein foods such as meat during mealtime.

Choose fresh plant foods and meat. Also, refrain from eating packed and processed foods, especially those that contain added phosphorus.

Check the phosphorus content of your food in the nutrition labels. Consult your nutritionist, dietician or physician.

PROTEIN

Protein is responsible for the growth and maintenance of all body tissues. It also plays an important role in fighting against opportunistic microorganisms, improving immunity and healing wounds. Protein is also one of the alternative sources of energy that can be utilized by your body. When protein is ingested and utilized by cells and tissues, waste products are formed. These wastes are normally filtered by the nephrons of the kidneys, turned into a form of urine and excreted from your body. When your kidneys are damaged, they fail to remove these protein wastes and they just accumulate in the blood. For people with chronic kidney disease, proper consumption of protein can be tricky. The amount of protein consumption varies at different stages of the disease. People with kidney problems need to consult their nephrologist or renal dietician about the recommended amount of protein for each stage of the disease.

FLUIDS

When you have end-stage kidney disease, you need to limit your daily fluid intake. This is because it can lead to fluid buildup in your body which is extremely dangerous. Common symptoms of too much fluid in the body include elevated blood pressure, swelling of the body and heart failure. Excess fluid can also build up around your lungs and cause chest pain, difficulty breathing and cardiac arrest. It is extremely important to follow the instructions of your nephrologist/nutritionist about proper fluid intake. Also, refrain from consuming foods that contain too much water, like soups, gelatin and some fruits/vegetables.

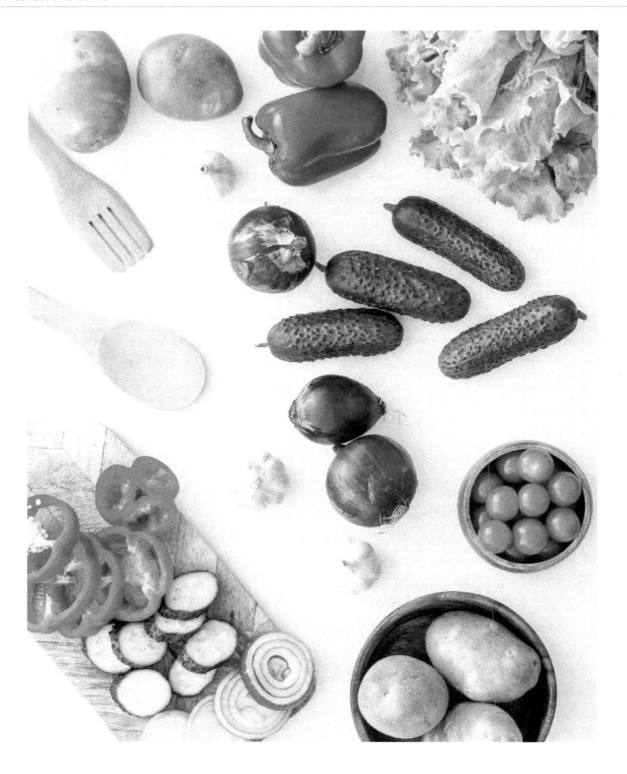

FOODS TO LIMIT/AVOID

People following a renal diet need should limit or avoid eating the following foods:

Dark-Colored Colas

Colas, especially the dark-colored ones, are high in calories, sugar and additives that contain phosphorus. This added phosphorus can be easily absorbed by the human body compared to natural phosphorus.

Canned Foods

Canned foods contain high amounts of sodium that can cause fluid retention in the body. People with kidney problems should avoid eating canned foods, especially when on a renal diet.

Avocados

People with kidney problems should avoid eating avocados because they contain high amounts of potassium that can be detrimental to their health. One cup of avocado contains almost 750 mg of potassium.

Brown Rice

Brown rice contains high amounts of potassium and phosphorus. 1 cup cooked brown rice contains 155 mg of potassium and 150 mg of phosphorus.

Bananas

Bananas contain high amounts of potassium and should be limited on a kidney diet.

Whole-Wheat Bread

Unlike white bread, whole-wheat bread contains high amounts of potassium and phosphorus. It also contains higher sodium levels that are bad for the kidneys.

Dairy Products

Dairy products are a rich source of potassium, phosphorus and protein and should be regulated on a kidney diet. Although milk contains high amounts of calcium, its high phosphorus content can cause weakening of the bones in people with kidney failure.

PROCESSED MEATS

Processed meats contain high amounts of salt and protein that can be harmful to the kidneys. These should be consumed in limited amounts on a kidney-friendly diet.

Apricots

Apricots are small, orange-colored fruits that are rich in Vitamins A and C. However, they are also a good source of potassium, which needs to be regulated on a renal diet.

Potatoes and Sweet Potatoes

Potatoes and sweet potatoes are high in potassium that can be harmful to one's health. Fortunately, boiling or double cooking potatoes can lower their potassium content by 50%.

Tomatoes

This high-potassium fruit needs to be regulated on a kidney-friendly diet. One cup of tomato sauce contains 750-900 mg of potassium. Dieters can replace the tomato sauce with a roasted pepper sauce, equally delicious but with less potassium.

Oranges and Orange Juice

While they are known for their Vitamin C content, oranges contain high amounts of potassium that should be limited on a kidney diet. One large-sized orange contains almost 300 mg of potassium while a cup 8-fluid-oz orange juice contains almost 500 mg of potassium.

Olives, Pickles and Relish

Processed olives, pickles and relish contain high amounts of sodium that can cause fluid retention. These foods should be limited to a renal diet.

Dates, Prunes and Raisins

Dried fruits like prunes, dates and raisins contain concentrated potassium that is 3-5 times higher than in their raw counterparts. This extremely high potassium can cause severe damage to the kidneys and can cause serious complications.

Spinach, Beet Greens and Swiss Chard

These leafy green vegetables are rich sources of potassium and other minerals. These veggies should be avoided or limited on a renal diet.

Chips, Crackers and Pretzels

These ready-to-eat snack foods contain relatively low amounts of healthy nutrients and high amounts of sodium (due to high salt content). Additionally, chips that are made from potatoes contain a significant amount of potassium that can be harmful to your kidneys.

Packaged, instant and Pre-Made Meals

Packaged, instant and pre-made meals are heavily processed foods and contain significantly high amounts of sodium. These foods also contain fewer amounts of helpful nutrients needed by the body. It is strongly advised to avoid consuming these foods while on a renal diet. Following a renal diet can be challenging and time-consuming. You need to constantly monitor your sodium, potassium and phosphorus intake to prevent further damage to your kidneys. You also need to monitor your fluid and protein intake to keep your kidneys safe and functioning. The foods mentioned above should be always avoided or limited while you are on a renal diet. If symptoms persist, seek help from medical professionals.

THE BEST FOODS ON A RENAL DIET

There are many foods that work well within the renal diet, and once you see the available variety, it will not seem as restrictive or difficult to follow. The key is focusing on the foods with a high level of nutrients, which makes it easier for the kidneys to process waste by not adding too much that the body needs to discard. Balance is a major factor in maintaining and improving long-term renal function.

Egg Whites

Eggs are high in protein and eating them in excess can put a lot of pressure on kidneys that are not functioning at their peak. There is the option of limiting the amount of eggs consumed to two per day, or using just the egg whites instead, as they provide the required nutrients without overtaxing the kidneys. Egg whites can be used in a variety of dishes just like whole eggs, such as omelets, scrambled eggs, soups and stir fry dishes. For people on dialysis, this is a healthier and safer option than using the whole egg.

Garlic

An excellent, vitamin-rich food for the immune system, garlic is a tasty substitute for salt in a variety of dishes. It acts as a significant source of vitamin C and B6, while aiding the kidneys in ridding the body of unwanted toxins. It's a great, healthy way to add flavor for skillet meals, pasta, soups and stews.

Berries

All berries are considered a good renal diet food due to their high level of fiber, antioxidants, and delicious taste, making them an easy option to include as a light snack or as an ingredient in smoothies, salads and light desserts. Just one handful of blueberries can provide almost one day's vitamin C requirement, as well as a boost of fiber, which is good for weight loss and maintenance.

Cabbage

For renal health, consider cabbage a superfood! Not only is this vegetable low in phosphorus, sodium and potassium, it's also an excellent source of minerals and vitamins that provide many of the required nutrients needed for a healthy, balanced diet. It's a good support for the digestive system and weight management, in addition to helping the kidneys. Cabbage is also a versatile food that can be used in a variety of dishes and cuisines, such as curries, baked cabbage rolls, soups, skillet meals and salads. All varieties of cabbage are excellent, from savoy to red cabbage, and just a moderate portion is needed to enjoy its nutritional benefits.

Bell Peppers

Flavorful and easy to enjoy both raw and cooked, bell peppers offer a good source of vitamin C, vitamin A, and fiber. Along with other kidney-friendly foods, they make the detoxification process much easier while boosting your body's nutrient level to prevent further health conditions and reduce existing deficiencies.

Onions

This nutritious and tasty vegetable is excellent as a companion to garlic in many dishes, or on its own. Like garlic, onions can provide flavor as an alternative to salt; plus they're a good source of vitamin C, vitamin B, manganese and fiber as well. Adding just one quarter or half of an onion is often enough for most meals, because of its strong, pungent flavor.

Macadamia Nuts

If you enjoy nuts and seeds as snacks, you many soon learn that many contain high amounts of phosphorus and should be avoided or limited as much as possible. Fortunately, macadamia nuts are an easier option to digest and process, as they contain much lower amounts of phosphorus and make an excellent substitute for other nuts. They are a good source of other nutrients, as well, such as vitamin B, copper, manganese, iron and healthy fats.

Pineapples

Unlike other fruits that are high in potassium, pineapple is an option that can be enjoyed more often than bananas and kiwis. Citrus fruits are generally high in potassium as well, so if you find yourself craving an orange or grapefruit, choose a pineapple instead. In addition to providing high levels of vitamin B and fiber, pineapples can reduce inflammation thanks to an enzyme called bromelain.

Mushrooms

In general, mushrooms are a safe, healthy option for the renal diet, especially the shiitake variety, which is high in nutrients such as selenium, vitamin B and manganese. They contain a moderate amount of plant-based protein, which is easier for your body to digest and use than animal proteins. Shiitake and portobello mushrooms are often used in vegan diets as a meat substitute, due to their texture and pleasant flavor.

THE CONNECTION BETWEEN DIET AND KIDNEY DISEASE

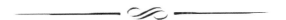

There is a distinct connection between the health and function of our kidneys and the way we eat. How we eat and the foods we choose have a significant impact on how well we feel and our overall wellbeing. Making changes to your diet is often necessary to guard against medical conditions, and while eating well can treat existing conditions, healthy food choices can also help prevent many other conditions from developing, including kidney disease. When we make changes to our diet, we often focus on the restrictions or foods we should avoid. While this is important, it's also vital to learn about the foods and nutrients we need in order to maintain good health and prevent disease. Consider the related conditions that contribute to high blood pressure and type-2 diabetes and the dietary changes often suggested to treat them and, in some successful cases, reverse the damage of these conditions. Dietary changes for the treatment and prevention of disease often focus on limiting salt, sugar and trans-fats from our food choices, while increasing minerals, protein and fiber, among other beneficial nutrients. The renal diet also focuses on eliminating, or at least limiting, the consumption of various ingredients to aid our kidneys to function better and to prevent further damage from occurring.

COMMON QUESTIONS & ANSWERS ABOUT THE RENAL DIET

Adapting to a new diet is a journey that brings about a lot of discoveries and questions about additional changes and options. The Renal Diet is no exception, and while it can be modified to suit custom preferences and tastes, you may have questions about the choices you make and how different foods and drinks affect your kidneys' health.

Q. Is a plant-based diet required to maximize the benefits of a renal diet?

A. A vegan diet is not a requirement of the renal diet, though it can be a great benefit if this is your preference. The most important aspect of eating well is to focus on fresh, plant-based foods, as they are easy to digest and contain significant amounts of nutrients. If you choose lean meats as part of your meal plan, be sure to include as many fresh fruits and vegetables as possible and limit the portions of animal protein with each serving, while increasing the amount of fiber and other nutrients.

Q. What happens if I find out that a specific food in my diet is too high in sodium, phosphorus, potassium or protein? Do I have to eliminate it completely, or may I indulge on occasion?

A. If your condition is severe, you may want to consult a doctor or specialist before making a firm decision. For most people, the occasional food choice such as a banana, which is high in potassium, is not going to have a negative impact and is often offset with many other health benefits within the renal diet guidelines, if followed closely. For this reason, there should be no adverse effects on your kidneys or health overall. In some cases, a dietitian or doctor may recommend certain foods outside of the renal diet if they notice a significant improvement in your kidneys and/ or to treat another ailment that could be related to kidney issues, such as high blood pressure or diabetes.

Q. What happens if I eat too much of the wrong foods and get off track. Is it too late to start the diet over again?

A. While it's important to adhere to this diet as much as possible, especially in more severe cases where renal function is low, don't get distracted with making the wrong food choices by switching back immediately. The odd "slip up" is expected, and anyone can make this error from time to time. The most important thing is to keep the basis of your food choices with your kidneys in mind, to avoid future errors and move towards a healthier lifestyle.

Q. Can I drink the occasional soda on the renal diet? Is it acceptable if the soda is sugar-free?

A. Drinking soda of any kind should be avoided, as the sugar content is so high (almost 30 grams of sugar in one can!). Artificial sweeteners in sugar-free sodas tend to be unhealthy and may cause unpleasant side effects of their own. If you want to enjoy a carbonated beverage, choose sparkling water with low sodium. Some of these drinks offer natural flavoring with little or no sugar, which makes them an excellent substitute.

Q. Is there a short list of foods to avoid?

A. Initially, when you begin this diet, it can be challenging to determine which foods are best to avoid. Unfortunately, while there is no short list, knowing which foods and types of meals to stay away from becomes easier in time. One of the first steps you can take is to avoid salty foods, which are known to be high in sodium and not a good fit for the renal diet. Foods high in protein should be limited as well, especially red meats. Plant-based sources of protein are much better for digestion, and easier on the kidneys. Foods high in phosphorus and potassium will become common once you familiarize yourself with them. In general, a better way to approach this diet is to focus on the foods you can have, as opposed to those you must limit or avoid.

Q. I've been following the renal diet for several months, but there haven't been any significant improvements to my kidneys. Does the renal diet work for everyone or just some people?

A. The answer to this question can vary dramatically, depending on the severity of the disease and stage of renal failure. In extreme cases where dialysis is involved, dietary changes may take much longer to have an impact than in situations where kidney disease has not progressed past the early stages and remains relatively easy to manage with diet. Other factors that may impact the variance in success or kidney improvement include the amount of excess weight, as it can take longer for some people to lose extra weight than others, glucose levels, and various stages of heart disease and/or type-2 diabetes. Given the number of variables that may affect your progress on the renal diet, always allow more time and keep a diary or journal to track any changes you notice. It may take longer than you expect, but by consistently following the meal plans and making better choices, you'll definitely see changes.

Q. How do I know if I'm eating too much protein or sodium? How can I avoid eating more phosphorus or potassium than my kidneys can handle, and how do I know when I've had too much?

A. Keeping a journal of your food options for meal planning is an ideal way to review your diet. Stay in regular contact with your doctor and share your meal plans, so they know exactly what you are eating on a daily basis. It may seem like a lot of work, but it's worthwhile until you become used to making informed decisions about the foods you eat. Every individual's circumstance is different: some people may have more leniency with the volume of protein and potassium they can consume, while those who use dialysis may need to restrict their choices further to ensure they can get the most out of the renal diet plan.

Q. Does the renal diet guarantee healthy kidneys if it is used as a preventative diet?

A. There is no guarantee that your kidneys will always function the same, and this refers to both healthy and impaired organs. Most people don't pay attention to the health of their kidneys until they are diagnosed with a condition, and only then are they faced with the decision to make dietary changes as soon as possible. Taking preventative measures doesn't necessarily require adherence to the renal diet, though aspects of this way of eating can be implemented into your diet to better support your kidneys while they are working well. If you have family or friends with kidney conditions, eating a renal-cautious diet with them and sharing meals is a good way to show your support while helping yourself at the same time. The best prevention is eating natural, whole foods, and focusing more on plantbased sources of nutrients. Reduce your animal proteins, and ensure you get the nutrients you need in moderation, without consuming too much sodium or protein. There is never a full guarantee that eating a well-balanced diet will prevent kidney disease completely, though it can be a great defense against renal disease and failure.

Q. Can the renal diet heal kidneys completely and restore their function to before they became infected?

A. Once damage to the kidneys occurs, it cannot be reversed; however, improvements can be made to ensure further damage is prevented and better function is restored, at least to an extent. For people who suffer from more advanced stages of renal disease, it is most important that the progress of the condition is arrested, so they can live longer and experience a better-quality life. Adhering to a renal diet is one way to ensure the kidneys get a "break" from toxins. Once you reach the stage of dialysis, it is vital to choose your meals as carefully as possible, as this becomes a requirement for the remainder of your life. If dietary and lifestyle changes can be successfully made prior to this stage, the prognosis is excellent, and you can lead a normal, productive life. Now more than ever, as we learn about the importance of kidney health, management of renal disease becomes a chronic condition with fewer complications, as long as you live a healthy lifestyle.

Q. Can medications interfere with the renal diet plan?

A. When prescribed a medication, either for your kidneys or another condition, always take the time to read about possible side effects, including food items to avoid. This may include some foods recommended on the renal diet. If in doubt, avoid any specific foods you may encounter reactions with as a result of the medication and consult with a pharmacist or doctor before proceeding. It's always best to avoid potential complications and play it safe before combining a potentially dangerous mix.

Q. Is kidney failure hereditary?

A. While there are some predisposed conditions that could lead to a higher chance of kidney disease or infection, there is no evidence to suggest kidney disease or renal failure is, in itself, hereditary. It is a fully preventable condition, and if you know of any kidney disease history in your family, you may be more likely to pay attention to the warning signs, especially early symptoms. Choosing your foods carefully and avoiding overeating and consuming processed foods will help you prevent kidney problems later in life.

UNDERSTANDING KIDNEY DISEASE

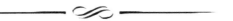

What is Chronic Kidney Disease (CKD)?

Chronic kidney disease (CKD) occurs when there are damaged kidneys or a kidney function decline for three months or more. There are five stages of evolution of a CRM according to the severity of the renal involvement or the degree of deterioration of its function.

Sometimes the kidney failure suddenly occurs. In this case, it is called an acute failure of the kidney. An injury, infection or something else may be the cause. Acute renal failure is often treated with urgency by dialysis for some time. Often, kidney function is recovered. Generally, this disease settles slowly and silently, but it progresses over the years. People with CKD do not necessarily go from stage 1 to stage 5 of the disease. Stage 5 of the disease is known under the name of end stage renal disease (ESRD) or kidney failure in the final stage.

It is important to know that the expressions terminal, final and ultimate mean the end of any function of the kidneys (kidneys working at less than 15% of their normal capacity) and not the end of your life. To stay alive at this stage of the disease, it is necessary to resort to dialysis or a kidney transplant. Dialysis and transplantation are known as renal replacement therapy (RRT).

This means that dialysis or the transplanted kidney will "supplement" or "replace" the sick kidneys and do their job.

Chronic kidney disease is a slow-progressing disease and does not cause the patient a lot of complaints in the initial stages. The group of diseases which are referred to as chronic kidney disease includes several kidney diseases in which the renal function decreases for several years or decades. With the help of timely diagnosis and treatment, we can slow down and even stop the progression of kidney disease.

In international studies of renal function in many people, it was found that almost every tenth kidney was found to have impaired kidney function to one degree or another.

With long-term diabetic kidney damage, many patients have increased blood pressure and need to be treated accordingly.

High blood pressure (hypertension, primary arterial hypertension) - during hypertension, blood pressure cannot be controlled, and it begins to exceed the limits of the norm (more than 140/90 mm Hg). If this condition is permanent, it can cause chronic kidney disease, brain stroke, or myocardial infarction.

Glomerulonephritis is a disease that occurs as a result of a breakdown in the immune system, during which the filtration function of the kidneys is disrupted by immune inflammation. The disease can affect only the kidneys or it can spread to the entire body (vacuities, lupus nephritis). Glomerulonephritis is often accompanied by high blood pressure.

Many other conditions can cause chronic kidney disease; for example hereditary diseases, such as polycystic kidney disease, occurring due to a large number of cysts appearing in the kidney over the years, which damage the functioning of the renal tissues and therefore develop renal failure. Other hereditary diseases of the kidneys which are much less common (Alport syndrome, Fabry disease, etc.) are caused by obstructions in the kidneys and urine excretion - such as congenital malformations of the ureter, kidney stones, tumors or enlargement of the prostate gland in men, repeated urinary tract infections or pyelonephritis.

What It Means to Have CKD?

It sounds scary when you get diagnosed with chronic kidney disease and you probably have a lot of questions. This disease can be managed very well. It takes some exploration, patience and time to see the big picture. Your first step to managing kidney disease is being able to understand it. Let's take a look at the role your kidneys play in your health, how your diet plays an important role in helping to manage kidney disease, and what happens when you develop kidney disease.

Once you have been diagnosed with CKD, it will be helpful to explore this disease and learn about some normal symptoms. A simple definition is a gradual loss of the function of your kidneys. Because our bodies constantly produce waste, our kidneys play a big role in removing these toxins and keeping our system working properly. Tests will be done to measure the level of waste in your blood and figure out how well your kidneys are working. Your doctor will be able to find out the filtration rate of your kidneys and figure out what stage of CKD you are in.

There are five stages that show how the kidneys function. Within the early stages, people won't experience any symptoms, and it is very easy to manage. Oftentimes, kidney disease isn't found until it becomes advanced. Most symptoms don't appear until the toxins build up in the body from the damage that has been done to the kidneys. This usually happens in the later stages. Changes in how you urinate, vomiting, nausea, swelling and itching could be caused by decreased ability to filtrate the toxins. This is why an early diagnosis that is critical to positive outcomes can come later when the disease has progressed.

There isn't a cure for CKD, but you can manage this disease. Making changes to your lifestyle and diet can slow down the progression and help you stay away from symptoms that normally start to show up later. These lifestyle changes can improve your total health and allow you to manage other conditions. Once you begin making changes to your daily food habits, you will see improvement in these conditions including diabetes and hypertension.

You can live a happy, healthy, and long life while managing CKD and making changes early can slow down the progression of this disease for years.

How the Kidneys Work

Our kidneys are bean-shaped filters that work in teams. They have a very important job since they keep our bodies stable. They use signals from the body like blood pressure and sodium content to help keep us hydrated and our blood pressure stable.

If the kidneys don't function right, there are numerous problems that could happen. When the filtration of these toxins becomes slow, these harmful chemicals can build up and cause other reactions within the body, like vomiting, nausea and rashes. When the kidney's functions continue to decrease, its ability to get rid of water and release hormones that control blood pressure can also be affected. Symptoms such as high blood pressure or retaining water in your feet might happen. With time having reduced kidney function could cause long-term health problems such as osteoporosis or anemia.

The kidneys work hard, so we have to protect them. They can filter around 120 to 150 quarts of blood each day. This will create between 1 and 2 quarts of urine that are made up of excess fluid and waste products.

What are the symptoms of chronic kidney disease?

If chronic kidney disease progresses, then the blood level of end products of metabolism increases; this in turn, is the cause of feeling unwell. Various health problems may occur, such as high blood pressure, anemia (anemia), bone disease, premature cardiovascular calcification, discoloration and change in the composition and volume of urine.

As the disease progresses, the main symptoms can be:

- Weakness, a feeling of weakness
- Trouble sleeping
- Lack of appetite
- Dry or itchy skin
- Muscle cramps, especially at night
- Swelling in the legs
- Swelling around the eyes, especially in the morning

Diagnosed with Chronic Kidney Disease

There are two simple tests that your family doctor can prescribe to diagnose a kidney disease.

Blood test

Glomerular filtration rate (GFR) and serum creatinine level. Creatinine is one of those end products of protein metabolism the level of which in the blood depends on age, gender, muscle mass, nutrition, physical activity, the foods taken before taking the sample (for example, a lot of meat was eaten) and some drugs. Creatinine is removed from the body through the kidneys, and if the kidneys slow down, the level of creatinine in the blood plasma increases. Determining the level of creatinine alone is not sufficient for the diagnosis of chronic kidney disease since its value begins to exceed the upper limit of the norm only when GFR is decreased by half. GFR is calculated using a formula that includes four parameters which are; the creatinine reading, age, gender and race of the patient. GFR shows the level at which the kidneys can filter. In the case of chronic kidney disease, the GFR indicator indicates the stage of the severity of kidney disease.

Ultrasound/ CT scan

These image-based tests can take clear images of your organs, particularly your kidneys, to see whether they look and function properly. This test can help doctors identify whether your kidneys are the right size and whether they have structural problems.

Kidney biopsy

This test is performed during sedation and is done by removing a tissue sample from the kidneys, which can indicate the health and damage of the organs.

Urine analysis

The content of albumin in the urine is determined; also, the values of albumin and creatinine in the urine are determined by each other. Albumin is a protein that usually enters the urine in minimal quantities. Even a small increase in the level of albumin in the urine may be an early sign of incipient kidney disease in some people, especially in those with diabetes and high blood pressure. In the case of normal kidney function, albumin in the urine should not be more than 3 mg/mmol (or 30 mg/g). If albumin excretion increases even more, then it already speaks of kidney disease.

Most Common Causes of Kidney Disease

Renal disease, according to experts, requires early diagnosis and targeted treatment to prevent or delay both a condition of acute or chronic renal failure and the appearance of cardiovascular complications to which it is often associated.

A fundamental role in alleviating the work of the already compromised kidneys is carried out by the diet which is, therefore, the first prevention. It must be studied with an expert nutritionist or a nephrologist in order to maintain or reach an ideal weight on the one hand and on the other, to reduce the intake of sodium (salt) and the consequent control of blood pressure and other substances (minerals), without creating malnutrition or nutritional deficiencies. Particular attention should also be paid to cholesterol, triglycerides and blood sugar levels.

Diabetes

We do know that diabetes is one of the leading causes of CKD. But we have yet to understand in detail why and how it can cause so much harm to the kidneys.

Time for a crash course in diabetes - What many may already know is that diabetes affects our body's insulin production rate. But what many may not know is the extent of damage that diabetes can cause to the kidneys.

Glomerulonephritis

The glomerulonephritis, or nephritis, appears when glomeruli, these little tiny filters used to purify the blood, deteriorate. There are several kinds of glomerulonephritis. Some are hereditary, while others occur as a result of certain diseases such as strep throat. The causes of most glomerulonephritis are not yet known. Some glomerulonephritis are cured without medical treatment, while others require prescription drugs. Some do not respond to any treatment and turn into chronic kidney disease. Some clues suggest that glomerulonephritis is due to a deficiency in the immune system of the body.

Autosomal Dominant Polycystic Disease

Often in their forties, people with the disease will need dialysis or a kidney transplant. But because the loss of kidney function is changing at a different pace, depending on the individual, the time between the onset of cysts and the need for dialysis varies widely. Since the disease is hereditary, people are advised to inform other family members to carry out the required tests as they too may be affected.

The Obstruction of the Urinary Tract

Any obstruction (or blockage) of the urinary tract may damage the kidneys. Obstructions can occur in the ureter or at the end of the bladder. Narrowing of the ureter at the superior or inferior level is sometimes due to congenital malformations, which sometimes leads to chronic kidney disease in children. In adults, increased prostate volume, kidney stones or tumors often obstruct the urinary tract.

Reflux Nephropathy

The reflux nephropathy is the new name of the former "chronic pyelonephritis."

Illegal Drugs

The use of illegal drugs can cause kidney damage. High-dose and long-term use of over-the-counter medications (without a prescription) can cause kidney damage.

Important: Beware of medications, including herbal remedies, sold without a prescription. It would be wiser to seek the advice of your doctor before buying them.

High Blood Pressure

An important thing to remember here is that high blood pressure can be both a cause and symptom of CKD, similar to the case of diabetes.

So, what exactly is blood pressure? People often throw the term around, but they are unable to pinpoint exactly what happens when the pressure in the blood increases.

Autoimmune Diseases

IgA nephropathy and lupus are two examples of autoimmune diseases that can lead to kidney diseases. But just what exactly are autoimmune diseases?

They are conditions where your immune system perceives your body as a threat and begins to attack it.

We all know that the immune system is like the defense force of our body. It is responsible for guiding our body's soldiers, known as white blood cells or WBCs. The immune system is responsible for fighting against foreign materials, such as viruses and bacteria. When the system senses these foreign bodies, various fighter cells, including the WBCs, are deployed in order to combat the threat.

Typically, your immune system is a self-learning system. This means that it is capable of understanding the threat and memorizing its features, behaviors and attack patterns. This is an important capability of the immune system since it allows the system to differentiate between our own cells and foreign cells. But when you have an autoimmune disease, your immune system suddenly considers certain parts of your body, such as your skin or joints, as foreign. It then proceeds to create antibodies that begin to attack these parts.

Kidney disease treatment options

There are various methods available for treating different kidney diseases, from the most complicated to the least complicated cases. Even though there are options made available to patients, one of the best ways to ensure you feel good internally, and to manage your stage effectively, is to follow a healthy and balanced lifestyle. Not only that, but one that is specifically tailored to your needs.

With that being said, it's also necessary to follow your own doctor's orders and take the necessary medication prescribed, to ensure your healthy journey towards either beating kidney disease and the issues you may experience related to kidney health or controlling the effects thereof. One of the most important reasons why kidney disease treatment is so important is that kidneys are prone to deteriorating. This not only disrupts the organs, but also the harmonic functioning and wellbeing of the entire body.

Your doctor will advise you how to treat kidney diseases properly after considering your blood sugar levels, blood pressure and cholesterol levels.

Prescribed medication

For chronic kidney disease patients, this can include angiotensin-converting enzyme (ACE) inhibitors, such as ramipril, lisinopril, as well as angiotensin receptor blockers (ARBs), like olmesartan and irbesartan. All of the mentioned medications are prescribed to kidney disease patients to manage their blood pressure and to slow down the disease. These are also prescribed to prevent kidney failure by supporting the necessary functions of the kidney. Sometimes, doctors may also prescribe cholesterol medication to reduce levels of cholesterol in the blood, such as simvastatin. In some cases, medication for inflammation and anemia can also be prescribed.

Diet and lifestyle changes

When you are diagnosed with a disease, especially one as serious as kidney disease, it is always recommended to change your diet and daily habits. Adopting diet rules and implementing the renal diet eating plan can prevent your kidney disease from getting worse and even prevent you from feeling sick every day. Since kidney disease has an effect on the entire body, there are plenty of ways, apart from your diet, to improve your habits and lifestyle.

Cutting back on salt (sodium), potassium, phosphorus, as we've already mentioned, as well as grains, low-fat dairy products, high-cholesterol foods and alcohol, you will significantly change the outcome of your health. Your doctor may also recommend you to treat diabetes with insulin injections, urge you to follow a healthier diet, like the renal diet for your health, quit smoking, increase your daily exercise levels and lose unhealthy weight.

Dialysis

In most cases, either hemodialysis, dialysis or peritoneal dialysis is recommended by doctors during stage four and stage five of kidney disease. It is only implemented when a patient's kidneys have reached a point of failure or are close to that point. Anyone that has reached these stages is required to receive dialysis until it is possible to conduct a kidney transplant.

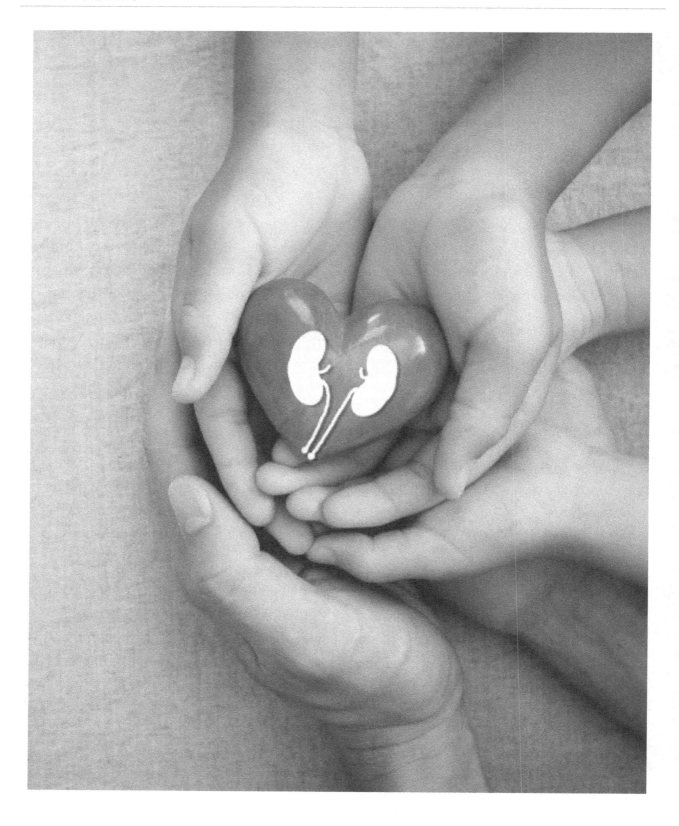

TIPS FOR HEALTHY KIDNEYS

A kidney disease diagnosis can seem devastating at first. The news may come as a shock for some people who may not have experienced any symptoms. It's important to remember that you can control your own progress and improvement through diet and lifestyle changes, even when a prognosis is serious. Taking steps to improve your health can make a significant effort to slow the progression of kidney disease and improve your quality of life.

You can do a lot of things if you want to keep your kidneys healthy and have them functioning properly. Here are certain tips that you can keep in mind for ensuring proper functioning of your kidneys.

Keep yourself hydrated

You should always make sure that you are sufficiently hydrated, but you shouldn't overdo it. No studies have shown that over-hydration is good for enhancing the performance of your kidneys. It is definitely good to drink sufficient water and you can drink around four to six glasses of water per day. Consuming more water than this wouldn't definitely help your kidneys perform better. In fact, it would just increase the stress on your kidneys.

Consume healthy foods

Your kidneys are capable of tolerating a wide variety of dietary habits and usually most of the kidney problems crop up from other existing medical conditions, like high blood pressure or diabetes. Because of this, it would be advisable to consume foods that will help you in regulating your weight and blood pressure. If you were able to prevent diabetes and even high blood pressure, then your kidneys would be healthy as well.

Exercise regularly

If you were already consuming foods that are healthy, then it would also make sense if you were exercising regularly. Because regular physical activity will prevent weight gain and also regulate your blood pressure. But you should be careful about the amount of time you exercise or how much you exercise, especially if you aren't used to exercising. Don't overexert yourself if you are just getting started, because this will just increase the pressure on your kidneys and can also result in the breaking down of your muscles.

Focus on Weight Loss

Losing weight is one of the most common reasons for going on a diet. It's also one of the best ways to treat kidney disease and prevent further damage. Carrying excess weight contributes to high toxicity levels in the body, by storing toxins instead of releasing them through the kidneys.

Commit

Be determined to change your lifestyle and habits. Your commitment to yourself and your motivation to follow through will help you manage your kidney disease. Keep in mind that the earlier this disease gets detected, the better you can treat it. There is a goal for your treatment: slowing down the disease and keeping it from getting any worse. This is one good thing about kidney disease: it lets you take control so you can manage it.

Understand Your Calorie Requirements

Each person's calorie requirements will be different, and it doesn't matter if they do or don't have CKD. If they do have CKD, picking the correct foods and eating the right number of calories will help their body. Calories give us the energy to function daily. They can help to slow the progression of kidney disease, keep a healthy weight, avoid losing muscle mass, prevent infections. Eating too many calories could cause weight gain, and that can put more of a burden on your kidneys. It is important that you get the correct number of calories. The number of calories for a person with CKD is about 60 to 70 calories per pound of body weight. If you weigh about 150 pounds, you need to consume around 2,000 calories per day.

Read Food Labels

It takes time to learn the renal diet and make it a part of your life. Lucky for you, all packaged foods come with nutrition labels along with an ingredient list. You need to read these labels so you can choose the right foods for your nutrition needs.

Portion Control

When you have kidney disease, controlling your portions is important. This doesn't mean you have to starve yourself. It doesn't matter what stage of CKD you are in but eating moderately is important when preserving your kidney health. The biggest part is making sure you don't feel deprived. You can enjoy many different foods as long as they are kidney-friendly and you don't overeat. When you cut back on foods that could harm your health and you are careful about what you eat, you are learning portion control. Make a habit of limiting specific foods and eating in moderation when following a kidney diet. It just takes having an informed game plan, resolve, and time.

Know Your Nutritional Needs

There isn't one diet plan that will be right for everybody who has kidney disease. What you are able to eat is going to change with time. It all depends on how well your kidneys function and factors such as being a diabetic. If you can work closely with your health team and constantly learn, you will be able to make healthy choices that will fit your needs. You can manage your disease and be successful.

Be careful when making use of supplements

If you are consuming any supplements or any other herbal remedies, then you should be mindful of the amount you are consuming. Consuming excessive amounts of vitamin supplements as well as any herbal extracts can prove to be harmful to the functioning of your kidneys. You should talk to your doctor before you start taking any supplements.

Quit smoking

Smoking causes damage to your blood vessels and this in turn will reduce the flow of blood to and in your kidneys. When the kidneys don't receive sufficient blood, they won't function like they are supposed to. Smoking also tends to increase your blood pressure and can also cause kidney cancer, apart from damaging your lungs.

Keep a track of your nutritional values

You should always keep track of what you are eating and also the serving size. You should keep a note of the nutritional values of the foods that you are consuming and discuss the same with your doctor.

Make use of meal-planning tools

It might be tiring and troublesome to plan your meals for one day, let alone planning for an entire week. This would feel like a daunting task. You should make use of the online meal-planning tools or mobile apps that can help you plan your meals for the entire week without much difficulty. When you know what you are supposed to consume on a daily basis, then you can stock up on the necessary groceries for the whole week.

Flavoring your meals without reaching out to the salt shaker

You should monitor the consumption of sodium if you want to follow the renal failure diet. A diet that is low in sodium will help in regulating your blood pressure and also will help you in fighting retention of fluids in your body. You can flavor your foods with spices, herbs and lemon juice instead!

Dining out

If you know that you will be going out to eat, then make sure that you have consumed as little sodium as possible during the rest of the day and opt for foods that contain less sodium when dining out.

CHAPTER 2 BREAKFAST

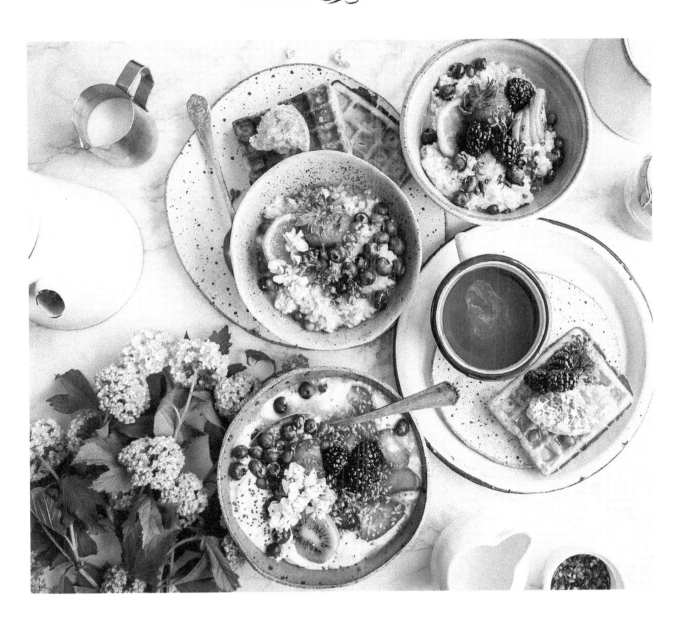

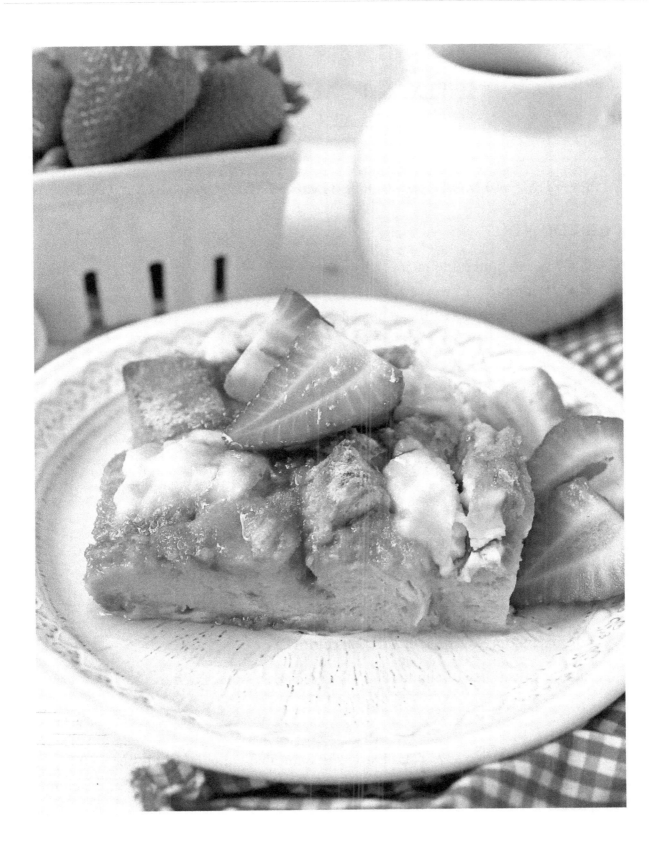

TEXAS TOAST CASSEROLE

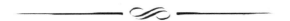

PREP TIME: 10 MINUTES | COOK TIME: 30 MINUTES | SERVINGS: 10

INGREDIENTS

- ½ cup butter, melted
- 1 cup brown Swerve
- 1 lb. Texas Toast bread, sliced
- 4 large eggs
- 1 ½ cup milk
- 1 tbsp vanilla extract
- 2 tbsps Swerve
- 2 tsps cinnamon
- Maple syrup for serving

DIRECTION

Layer a 9x13-inch baking pan with cooking spray.

Spread the bread slices at the bottom of the prepared pan.

Whisk the eggs with the remaining ingredients in a mixer.

Pour this mixture over the bread slices evenly.

Bake the bread for 30 minutes at 350 degrees F in a preheated oven.

Serve.

Nutrition: Calories 332, Total Fat 13.7g, Saturated Fat 6.9g, Cholesterol 102mg, Sodium 350mg, Carbohydrates 22.6g, Dietary Fiber 2g, Sugars 6g, Protein 7.4g, Calcium 143mg, Phosphorus 186mg, Potassium 74mg

ZUCCHINI BREAD

PREP TIME: 10 MINUTES | COOK TIME: 1 HOUR | SERVINGS: 16

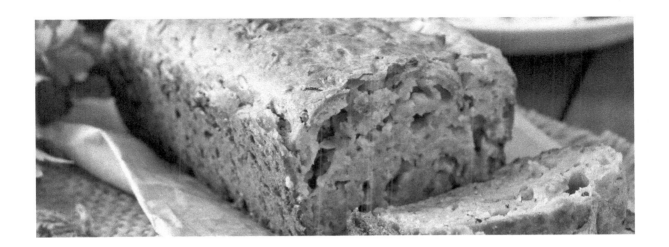

INGREDIENTS

- 3 eggs
- 1 ½ cups Swerve
- 1 cup apple sauce
- 2 cups zucchini, shredded
- 1 tsp vanilla
- 2 cups flour
- ¼ tsp baking powder
- 1 tsp baking soda
- 1 tsp cinnamon
- ½ tsp ginger
- 1 cup unsalted nuts, chopped

DIRECTION

Thoroughly whisk the eggs with the zucchini, apple sauce, and the rest of the ingredients in a bowl. Once mixed evenly, spread the mixture in a loaf pan. Bake it for 1 hour at 375 degrees F in a preheated oven. Slice and serve.

NUTRITION

Calories 200, Total Fat 5.4g, Saturated Fat 0.9g, Cholesterol 31mg, Sodium 94mg, Carbohydrates 26.9g, Dietary Fiber 1.6g, Sugars 16.3g, Protein 4.4g, Calcium 20mg, Phosphorus 212mg, Potassium 137mg

GARLIC MAYO BREAD

PREP TIME: 10 MINUTES | COOK TIME: 5 MINUTES | SERVINGS: 16

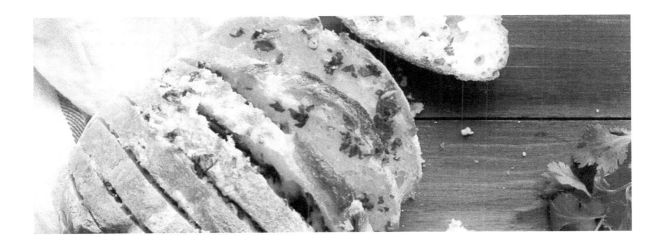

INGREDIENTS

- 3 tbsps vegetable oil
- 4 cloves garlic, minced
- 2 tsps paprika Dash cayenne pepper
- 1 tsp lemon juice
- 2 tbsps Parmesan cheese, grated
- 3/4 cup mayonnaise
- 1 loaf (1 lb.) French bread, sliced
- 1 tsp Italian herbs

DIRECTION

Mix the garlic with the oil in a small bowl and leave it overnight. Discard the garlic from the bowl and keep the garlic-infused oil. Mix the garlic-oil with cayenne, paprika, lemon juice, mayonnaise, and Parmesan. Place the bread slices in a baking tray lined with parchment paper. Top these slices with the mayonnaise mixture and drizzle the Italian herbs on top. Broil these slices for 5 minutes until golden brown. Serve warm.

NUTRITION

Calories 217, Total Fat 7.9g, Saturated Fat 1.8g, Cholesterol 5mg, Sodium 423mg, Carbohydrate 30.3g, Dietary Fiber 1.3g, Sugars 2g, Protein 7g, Calcium 56mg, Phosphorus 347mg, Potassium 72mg

CHIA PUDDING

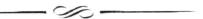

PREP TIME: 10 MINUTES | COOK TIME: 30 MINUTES | SERVINGS: 2

INGREDIENTS

- ½ cup raspberries
- 2 tsps maple syrup
- 1 ½ cup Plain yogurt
- ¼ tsp ground cardamom
- 1/3 cup Chia seeds, dried

DIRECTION

- Mix together Plain yogurt with maple syrup and ground cardamom.
- Add Chia seeds. Stir it gently.
- Put the yogurt in the serving glasses and top with the raspberries.
- Refrigerate the breakfast for at least 30 minutes or overnight.

NUTRITION: CALORIES 303, FAT 11.2G, FIBER 11.8G, CARBS 33.2G, PROTEIN 15.5G

PARMESAN ZUCCHINI FRITTATA

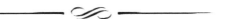

PREP TIME: 10 MINUTES | COOK TIME: 35 MINUTES | SERVINGS: 6

INGREDIENTS

- 1 tbsp olive oil
- 1 cup yellow onion, sliced
- 3 cups zucchini, chopped
- ½ cup Parmesan cheese, grated
- 8 large eggs
- ½ tsp black pepper
- 1/8 tsp paprika
- 3 tbsps parsley, chopped

DIRECTION

Toss the zucchinis with the onion, parsley, and all the other ingredients in a large bowl.

Pour this zucchini-garlic mixture in an 11x7-inch pan and spread it evenly.

Bake the zucchini casserole for approximately 35 minutes at 350 degrees F.

Cut in slices and serve.

NUTRITION: Calories 142, Total Fat 9.7g, Saturated Fat 2.8g, Cholesterol 250mg, Sodium 123mg, Carbohydrates 4.7g, Dietary Fiber 1.3g, Sugars 2.4g, Protein 10.2g, Calcium 73mg, Phosphorus 375mg, Potassium 286mg

APPLE CINNAMON RINGS

PREP TIME: 10 MINUTES | COOK TIME: 20 MINUTES | SERVINGS: 6

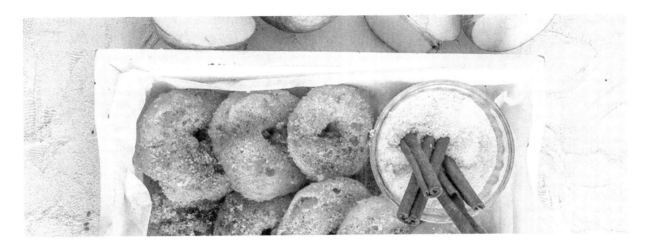

INGREDIENTS

- 4 large apples, cut in rings
- 1 cup flour
- ¼ tsp baking powder
- 1 tsp stevia
- ¼ tsp cinnamon
- 1 large egg, beaten
- 1 cup milk
- Vegetable oil, for frying Cinnamon Topping:
- 1/3 cup of brown Swerve
- 2 tsps cinnamon

DIRECTION

Begin by mixing the flour with the baking powder, cinnamon and stevia in a bowl. Whisk the egg with the milk in a bowl. Stir in the dry flour mixture and mix well until it makes a smooth batter. Pour oil into a wok to deep fry the rings and heat it up to 375 degrees F. First, dip the apple in the flour batter and deep fry until golden brown. Transfer the apple rings on a tray lined with paper towel. Drizzle the cinnamon and Swerve topping over the slices. Serve fresh in the morning.

NUTRITION

Calories 166, Total Fat 1.7g, Saturated Fat 0.5g, Cholesterol 33mg, Sodium 55mg, Carbohydrates 13.1g, Dietary Fiber 1.9g, Sugars 6.9g, Protein 4.7g, Calcium 65mg, Phosphorus 241mg, Potassium 197mg

YOGURT BULGUR

PREP TIME: 10 MINUTES | COOK TIME: 15 MINUTES | SERVINGS: 3

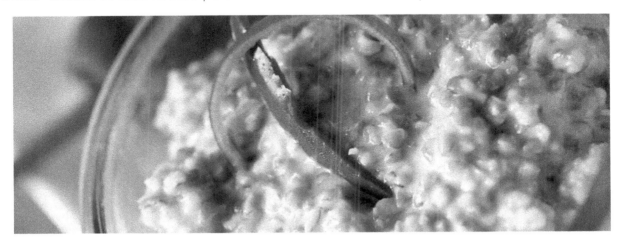

INGREDIENTS

- 1 cup bulgur
- 2 cups Greek yogurt
- 1 ½ cup water
- ½ tsp salt
- 1 tsp olive oil

DIRECTION

Pour olive oil in the saucepan and add bulgur. Roast it over the medium heat for 2-3 minutes. Stir it from time to time. After this, add salt and water. Close the lid and cook bulgur for 15 minutes over the medium heat. Then chill the cooked bulgur well and combine it with Greek yogurt. Stir it carefully. Transfer the cooked meal into the serving plates. The yogurt bulgur tastes best when it is cold.

NUTRITION

CALORIES 274, FAT 4.9G, FIBER 8.5G, CARBS 40.8G, PROTEIN 19.2G

DEVILED EGGS

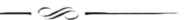

PREP TIME: 5 MINUTES | COOK TIME: 20 MINUTES | SERVINGS: 3

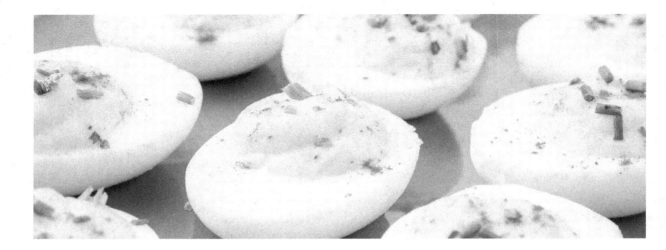

INGREDIENTS

- 4 hardboiled eggs
- 1 tbsp chopped onion
- ½ tbsp vinegar
- ½ tbsp dry mustard
- 2 tbsps mayonnaise Pepper to taste pinch of paprika

DIRECTION

Mash the yolk with a fork and mix to taste with the onion, vinegar, dry mustard, mayonnaise and pepper. Fill the eggs by filling them lightly. Sprinkle with paprika.

NUTRITION

Calories 96kcal Potassium 103mg Sodium 370mg Phosphorus 93mg Protein 7g

GOAT CHEESE OMELET

PREP TIME: 10 MINUTES | COOK TIME: 25 MINUTES | SERVINGS: 8

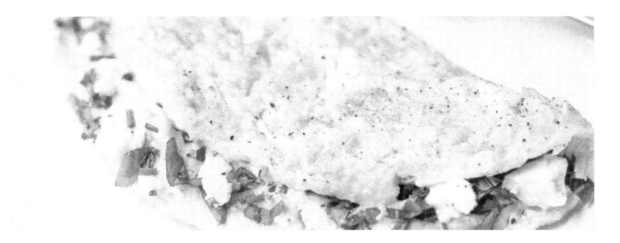

INGREDIENTS

- 8 eggs, beaten
- 6 oz Goat cheese, crumbled
- ½ tsp salt
- 3 tbsps sour cream
- 1 tsp butter
- ½ tsp canola oil
- ¼ tsp sage
- ¼ tsp dried oregano
- 1 tsp chives, chopped

DIRECTION

Put butter in the skillet. Add canola oil and preheat the mixture until it is homogenous. Meanwhile, combine salt, sour cream, sage, dried oregano, and chives in a mixing bowl. Add eggs and stir the mixture carefully with a spoon/fork. Pour the egg mixture in the skillet with butter-oil liquid. Sprinkle the omelet with goat cheese and close the lid. Cook the breakfast for 20 minutes over a low heat. The cooked omelet should be solid. Slice it and transfer to the plates.

NUTRITION

CALORIES 176, FAT 13.7G, FIBER 0G, CARBS 0G, PROTEIN 12.2G

BREAKFAST POTATO LATKES WITH SPINACH

PREP TIME: 10 MINUTES | COOK TIME: 6 MINUTES | SERVINGS: 4

INGREDIENTS

- 2 potatoes, peeled
- ½ onion, diced
- ½ cup spinach, chopped
- 2 eggs, beaten
- ½ tsp salt
- ½ tsp ground black pepper
- 1 tsp olive oil

DIRECTION

Grate the potato and mix it with chopped spinach, diced onion, salt and ground black pepper. Add eggs and stir until homogenous. Then pour olive oil in the skillet and preheat it well.

Make the medium latkes with 2 spoons and transfer them in the preheated oil. Roast the latkes for 3 minutes on each side or until they are golden brown. Dry the cooked latkes with the help of the paper towel if needed.

NUTRITION:

CALORIES 122, FAT 3.5G, FIBER 3G, CARBS 18.5G, PROTEIN 4.9G

OLIVE BREAD

———— ⤲ ————

PREP TIME: 20 MINUTES | COOK TIME: 50 MINUTES | SERVINGS: 6

INGREDIENTS

- 1 cup black olives, pitted, chopped
- 1 tbsp olive oil
- ½ tsp fresh yeast
- ½ cup milk, preheated
- ½ tsp salt
- 1 tsp baking powder
- 2 cup wheat flour, whole grain
- 2 eggs, beaten
- 1 tsp butter, melted
- 1 tsp sugar

DIRECTION

In a big bowl, combine fresh yeast, sugar and milk. Stir until yeast is dissolved. Then add salt, baking powder, butter and eggs. Stir the dough mixture until homogenous and add 1 cup of wheat flour. Mix until smooth. Add olives and remaining flour. Knead the non-sticky dough. Transfer the dough into the non-sticky dough mold. Bake the bread for 50 minutes at 350 F. Check if the bread is cooked by poking it with a toothpick. If the toothpick is dry, the bread is cooked. Remove the bread from the oven and let it chill for 10-15 minutes. Remove it from the loaf mold and slice.

NUTRITION:

CALORIES 238, FAT 7.7G, FIBER 1.9G, CARBS 35.5G, PROTEIN 7.2G

VANILLA SCONES

PREP TIME: 20 MINUTES | COOK TIME: 10 MINUTES | SERVINGS: 4

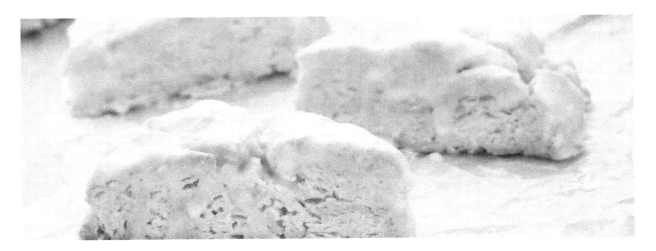

INGREDIENTS

- ½ cup wheat flour, whole grain
- 1 tsp baking powder
- 1 tbsp butter, melted
- 1 tsp vanilla extract
- 1 egg, beaten
- ¾ tsp salt
- 3 tbsps milk
- 1 tsp vanilla sugar

DIRECTION

In a mixing bowl, combine wheat flour, baking powder, butter, vanilla extract and egg.

Add salt and knead the soft and non-sticky dough. Add more flour if needed. Then make a log from the dough and cut it into triangles. Line the tray with baking paper. Arrange the dough triangles on the baking paper and transfer in the oven preheated to 360F. Cook the scones for 10 minutes or until they are light brown. After this, chill the scones, brush them with milk and sprinkle with vanilla sugar.

NUTRITION

CALORIES 112, FAT 4.4G, FIBER 0.5G, CARBS 14.3G, PROTEIN 3.4G

YUFKA PIES

PREP TIME: 15 MINUTES | COOK TIME: 20 MINUTES | SERVINGS: 6

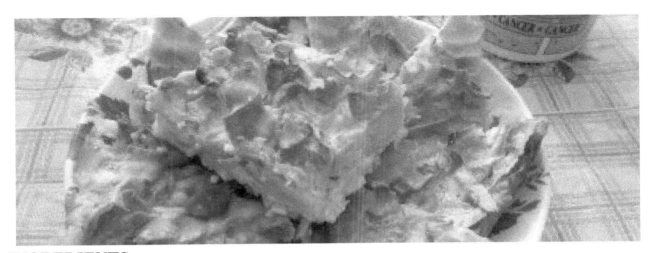

INGREDIENTS

- 7 oz yufka dough/phyllo dough
- 1 cup Cheddar cheese, shredded
- 1 cup fresh cilantro, chopped
- 2 eggs, beaten
- 1 tsp paprika
- ¼ tsp chili flakes
- ½ tsp salt
- 2 tbsps sour cream
- 1 tsp olive oil

DIRECTION

In the mixing bowl, combine together sour cream, salt, chili flakes, paprika and beaten eggs. Brush the springform pan with olive oil. Place ¼ of all yufka dough in the pan and sprinkle it with ¼ of the egg mixture. Add a ¼ cup of cheese and ¼ cup of cilantro. Cover the mixture with 1/3 of remaining yufka dough and repeat the all the steps again. You should get 4 layers. Cut the yufka mixture into 6 pies and bake at 360F for 20 minutes. The cooked pies should have a golden-brown color.

NUTRITION

CALORIES 213, FAT 11.4G, FIBER 0.8G, CARBS 18.2G, PROTEIN 9.1G

CHERRY TOMATOES AND FETA FRITATTA

PREP TIME: 10 MINUTES | COOK TIME: 25 MINUTES | SERVINGS: 4

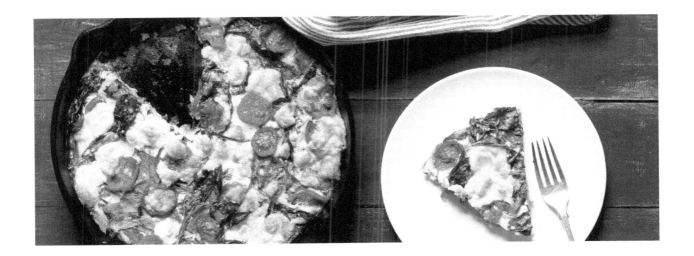

INGREDIENTS

- 4 eggs, beaten
- 1/3 cup cherry tomatoes
- 2 oz Feta cheese, crumbled
- 1 tsp butter
- 1 tsp fresh parsley, chopped
- ½ tsp salt
- ½ tsp dried oregano

DIRECTION

Cut the cherry tomatoes into halves. Then spread the round springform pan with butter.

Arrange the cherry tomato halves in the pan in one layer. Then add a layer of Feta cheese. In a mixing bowl, mix beaten eggs, dried oregano, salt and parsley. Pour the egg mixture over the cheese. Preheat the oven to 360F. Put the pan with frittata in the oven and cook it for 25 minutes at 355F

NUTRITION

CALORIES 112, FAT 4.4G, FIBER 0.5G, CARBS 14.3G, PROTEIN 3.4G

EGG WHITE SCRAMBLE

PREP TIME: 10 MINUTES | COOK TIME: 6 MINUTES | SERVINGS: 4

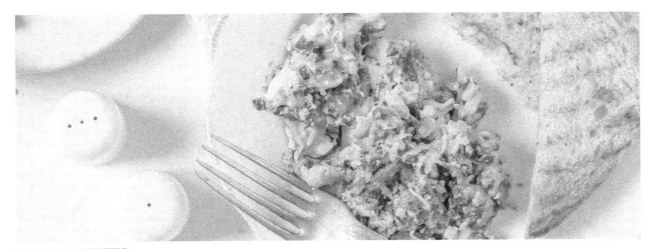

INGREDIENTS

- 1 tsp almond butter
- 4 egg whites
- ¼ tsp salt
- ½ tsp paprika
- 2 tbsps heavy cream

DIRECTION

Whisk the egg whites gently and add heavy cream. Put the almond butter in a skillet and melt it. Then add the egg white mixture. Sprinkle it with salt and cook for 2 minutes over medium heat. After this, scramble the egg whites with a fork or spatula and sprinkle with paprika. Cook the scrambled egg whites for 3 more minutes. Transfer the meal onto serving plates.

NUTRITION: CALORIES 68, FAT 5.1G, FIBER 0.5G, CARBS 1.3G, PROTEIN 4.6G

CHAPTER 3 APPETIZERS

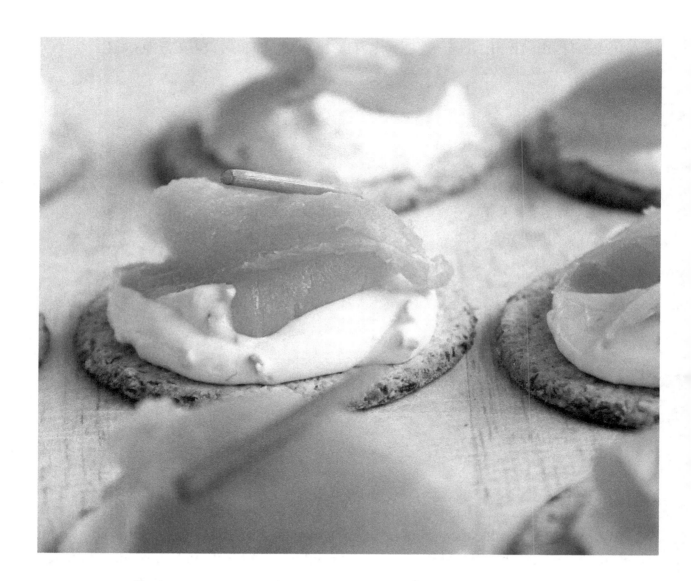

APPETIZERS

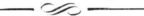

63. CREAMY GRAPE SALAD

64. AVOCADO CILANTRO DETOX DRESSING

65. GOLDEN TURMERIC SAUCE

66. GINGER SESAME SAUCE

67. CREAMY TURMERIC DRESSING

68. DIJON MUSTARD VINAIGRETTE

69. ANTI-I N FLAMMATORY CAESAR DRESSING

70. FRESH TOMATO VINAIGRETTE

71. GOLDEN TURMERIC TAHINI SAUCE

72. SWEET BALSAMIC DRESSING

73. HEALTHY TERIYAKI SAUCE

74. YOGURT GARLIC SAUCE

75. CHUNKY TOMATO SAUCE

76. CITRUS SALAD SAUCE

77. ANTI-I N FLAMMATORY APPLESAUCE

78. POPPY SEED-LEMON DRESSING ON WINTER FRUIT SALAD

79. JANE'S APPLE SALAD

APPETIZERS

80. HEART HEALTHY CHICKEN SALAD

81. SPINACH AND CRANBERRY SALAD

82. GREEN PEA SALAD

83. QUINOA, CILANTRO AND CRANBERRY SALAD

84. WILD RICE SALAD

85. TUNA CAPRESE SALAD

CREAMY GRAPE SALAD

———— ∽ ————

PREP TIME: 10 MINUTES | COOK TIME: 15 MINUTES | SERVINGS: 6

INGREDIENTS

- 6c. grapes
- 8 oz. Cream cheese
- 8 oz. sour cream, softened at room temperature
- ½ tsp. Granulated sugar
- ½ tsp vanilla extract

DIRECTION

Wash the grapes. In a large bowl, combine the cream cheese, sour cream and vanilla extract, then add the powdered sugar. Add the grapes and mix until homogeneous. Let cool in the cold and serve.

NUTRITION:

CALORIES 182KCAL SODIUM 197MG POTASSIUM 77MG PHOSPHORUS 57MG PROTEIN 2G

AVOCADO CILANTRO DETOX DRESSING

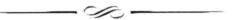

PREP TIME: 5 MINUTES | COOK TIME: 0 MINUTES | SERVINGS: 3

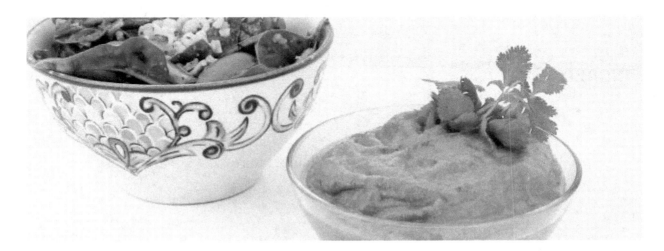

INGREDIENTS

- 5 tbsps lemon juice, freshly squeezed
- 1 clove of garlic, chopped
- 1 avocado, pitted and flesh scooped out
- 1 bunch cilantro, chopped
- ¼ tsp salt
- ¼ cup water

DIRECTION

Place all ingredients in a food processor and pulse until well combined. Pulse until creamy. Place in a lidded container and store in the fridge until ready to use. Use on salads and sandwiches.

NUTRITION :Calories 114, Total Fat 10g, Saturated Fat 1g, Total Carbs 8g, Net Carbs 3g, Protein 2g, Sugar: 2g, Fiber 5 G, Sodium 5mg, Potassium 355mg

GOLDEN TURMERIC SAUCE

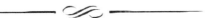

PREP TIME: 10 MINUTES | COOK TIME: 15 MINUTES | SERVINGS: 4

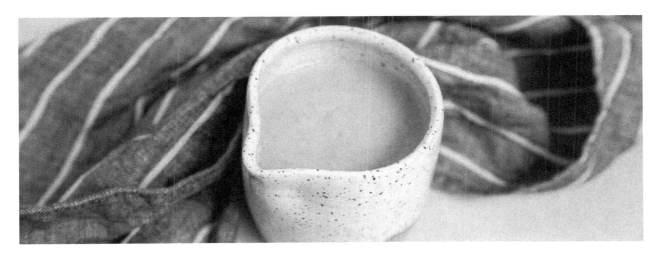

INGREDIENTS

- 2 tbsps coconut oil
- 1 onion, chopped
- 2-inch piece ginger, peeled and minced
- 2 cloves of garlic, minced
- 2 cups white sweet potato, cubed
- 2 tbsps turmeric powder
- ½ tsp ginger powder
- ¼ tsp cinnamon powder
- 2 cups coconut milk
- Juice from 1 lemon, freshly squeezed
- 1 cup water
- 1 ½ tsp salt

DIRECTION

Heat oil in a saucepan over medium flame. Sauté the onion, ginger and garlic until fragrant. Add in the sweet potatoes, turmeric powder, ginger powder and cinnamon powder. Pour in water and season with salt. Bring to a boil for 10 minutes. Once the potatoes are soft, place in a blender pulse until smooth. Return the mixture into the saucepan. Turn on the stove. Add in the coconut milk and lemon juice. Allow to simmer for 5 minutes. Store in lidded containers and put inside the fridge until ready to use.

NUTRITION:

Calories 172, Total Fat 11g, Saturated Fat 2g, Total Carbs 15g, Net Carbs 12g, Protein 5g, Sugar: 8g, Fiber: 3g, Sodium: 36mg, Potassium 408mg

GINGER SESAME SAUCE

Preparation Time: 5 minutes Cooking Time: 0 minutes Serving: 6

INGREDIENTS:

- ½ cup olive oil
- ¼ cup sesame oil
- 1/3 cup rice wine vinegar
- 1 tbsp fresh ginger
- 1 tbsp sesame seeds

DIRECTIONS:

Place all ingredients in a food processor.

Pulse until a smooth paste is formed.

Place in containers and store in the fridge until ready to use.

NUTRITION:

Calories250, Total Fat 28g, Saturated Fat 4g, Total Carbs 0.2g, Net Carbs 0.1g, Protein 0.3g, Sugar 0.01g, Fiber 0.1g, Sodium 2mg, Potassium 10 mg

CREAMY TURMERIC DRESSING

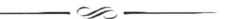

Preparation Time: 5 minutes Cooking Time: 0 minutes Serving: 6

INGREDIENTS

- ½ cup tahini
- ½ cup olive oil
- 2 tbsps lemon juice
- 2 tsps honey
- Salt to taste
- a dash of black pepper

DIRECTIONS

Mix all ingredients in a bowl until creamy and smooth.

Store in lidded containers.

Put in the fridge until ready to use.

NUTRITION

Calories 286, Total Fat 29g, Saturated Fat 4g, Total Carbs 7g, Net Carbs 5g, Protein 4g, Sugar 2g, Fiber 2 g, Sodium 24mg, Potassium 89mg

Dijon Mustard Vinaigrette

Preparation Time: 5 minutes Cooking Time: 0 minutes Serving: 6

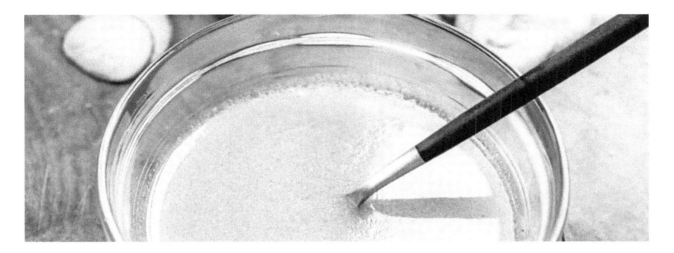

INGREDIENTS

- ¾ cup olive oil
- ¼ cup apple cider vinegar
- 3 tbsps Dijon mustard
- 2 shallots, quartered
- 1 garlic clove, chopped
- A handful of parsley, chopped

DIRECTIONS

Place all ingredients in a food processor.

Pulse until smooth.

Place in containers and store in the fridge until ready to use.

NUTRITION

Calories 252, Total Fat 27g, Saturated Fat 4g, Total Carbs 2g, Net Carbs 1.3g, Protein 0.6g, Sugar 1g, Fiber: 0.7g, Sodium 80 mg, Potassium 93mg

ANTI-INFLAMMATORY CAESAR DRESSING

Preparation Time: 5 minutes Cooking Time: 0 minutes Serving: 6

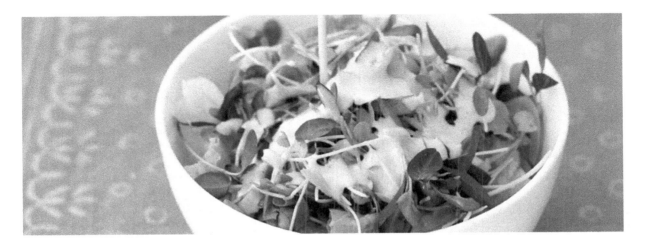

INGREDIENTS

- ½ cup cashew nuts, soaked in water then drained
- 1/3 cup fresh lemon juice
- 1 clove of garlic, minced
- 1 tbsp Dijon mustard
- 1 tbsp anchovy paste
- 2 tbsp extra-virgin olive oil
- ½ cup plain Greek yogurt

DIRECTIONS

Place all ingredients in a food processor.

Pulse until a smooth paste is formed.

Place in containers and store in the fridge until ready to use.

NUTRITION

Calories 96, Total Fat 7g, Saturated Fat 1.2g, Total Carbs 5g, Net Carbs 4.5g, Protein 4g, Sugar 1g, Fiber 0.5g, Sodium 113mg, Potassium 132mg

Fresh Tomato Vinaigrette

Preparation Time: 5 minutes Cooking Time: 0 minutes Serving: 5

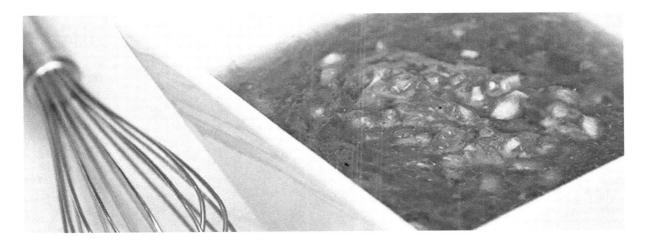

INGREDIENTS

- 1 fresh tomato, chopped
- ¾ cup olive oil
- ¼ cup apple cider vinegar
- 1 clove of garlic, chopped
- ½ tsp dried oregano
- Salt and pepper to taste

DIRECTIONS

Place all ingredients in a food processor.

Pulse until a smooth paste is formed.

Place in containers and store in the fridge until ready to use.

NUTRITION

Calories 298, Total Fat 32g, Saturated Fat 5g, Total Carbs 2g, Net Carbs g, Protein 0.2g, Sugar 2g, Fiber 0.4g, Sodium 3mg, Potassium 75mg

Golden Turmeric Tahini Sauce

Preparation Time: 5 minutes Cooking Time: 0 minutes Serving: 6

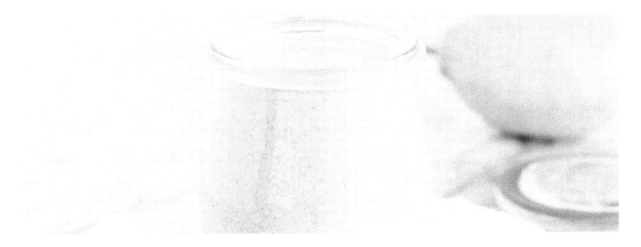

INGREDIENTS

- ¼ cup tahini
- ¼ cup lemon juice
- 1 tbsp olive oil
- 1 tbsp nutritional yeast
- ½ tbsp maple syrup
- ¼ tsp ground turmeric
- A pinch of cayenne pepper
- 2 tbsps water
- ¼ tsp salt
- ¼ tsp black pepper

DIRECTIONS

Place all ingredients in a food processor.

Pulse until a smooth paste is formed.

Place in containers and store in the fridge until ready to use.

NUTRITION

Calories 71, Total Fat 6g, Saturated Fat 1g, Total Carbs4 g, Net Carbs 3g, Protein 2g, Sugar 1g, Fiber 1g, Sodium 56mg, Potassium 341mg

SWEET BALSAMIC DRESSING

Preparation Time: 5 minutes Cooking Time: 0 minutes Serving: 5

INGREDIENTS:

- 1 cup olive oil
- ½ cup balsamic vinegar
- 2 tsps raw honey
- 2 tsps mustard
- 2 cloves of garlic, minced
- Salt and pepper to taste

DIRECTIONS:

Combine all ingredients in a blender and pulse until the mixture becomes smooth.

Place in contains until ready to use.

NUTRITION:

Calories 416, Total Fat 43g, Saturated Fat 6g, Total Carbs 7g, Net Carbs 6.9g, Protein 0.3g, Sugar 6 g, Fiber 0.1g, Sodium 29mg, Potassium 38mg

HEALTHY TERIYAKI SAUCE

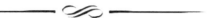

Preparation Time: 5 minutes Cooking Time: 8 minutes Serving: 6

INGREDIENTS:

- ½ cup reduced-sodium tamari
- ¼ cup pitted dates, pulsed until smooth
- 1 ½ tsps minced garlic
- 1 ½ tsps minced ginger
- 1 tbsp blackstrap molasses
- 2 tbsps sweet rice cooking wine
- 2 tsps arrowroot powder + 2 tsps water
- ¼ cup water

DIRECTIONS:

Place all ingredients except for the arrowroot slurry in a saucepan.

Turn on the heat and bring to a simmer for 5 minutes over medium flame.

Add in the arrowroot slurry and continue cooking for another 3 minutes or until the sauce thickens.

Place in containers and store in the fridge.

NUTRITION:

Calories 236, Total Fat 11g, Saturated Fat 2g, Total Carbs 31g, Net Carbs 29g, Protein 7g, Sugar 11g, Fiber 2g, Sodium 245mg, Potassium 274mg

YOGURT GARLIC SAUCE

Preparation Time: 5 minutes Cooking Time: 0 minutes Serving: 4

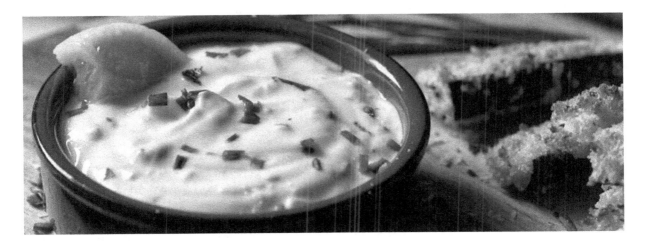

INGREDIENTS:

- 1 cup yogurt
- 1 clove of garlic, minced
- 1/3 cup parsley, finely chopped
- Juice from ½ lemon

DIRECTIONS:

Place all ingredients in a bowl.

Whisk to combine everything.

Put in a container with lid and store in the fridge until ready to use.

NUTRITION:

Calories 42, Total Fat 2g, Saturated Fat 1g, Total Carbs 4g, Net Carbs 3.8g, Protein 2g, Sugar 3g, Fiber 0.2 g, Sodium 31mg, Potassium 132mg

Chunky Tomato Sauce

Preparation Time: 5 minutes Cooking Time: 15 minutes Serving: 6

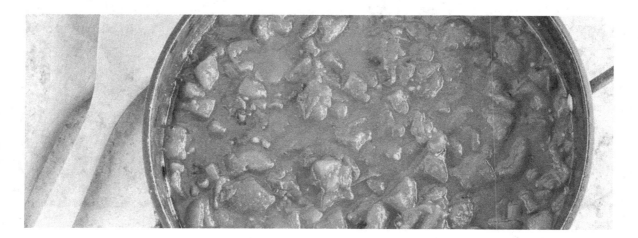

INGREDIENTS:

- ¼ cup extra virgin olive oil
- 2 onions, chopped
- 5 cloves of garlic, minced
- 2 red bell peppers, chopped
- ½ cup sliced Portobello mushrooms
- 3 cups diced tomatoes
- 1 tsp dried oregano
- 2 tsps honey
- 2 tsps balsamic vinegar
- 1 tsp dried basil
- ½ cup fresh spinach, chopped
- salt and pepper to taste

DIRECTIONS:

In a heavy pan, heat oil over medium flame.

Stir in the onions, garlic and bell pepper until fragrant.

Add in the mushrooms, tomatoes, oregano, honey, balsamic vinegar and basil. Season with salt and pepper to taste.

Close the lid and bring to a simmer for 10 minutes until the tomatoes have wilted.

Add in the spinach last and cook for another 5 minutes.

Place in containers and store in the fridge until ready to use.

NUTRITION:

Calories 86, Total Fat 4g, Saturated Fat 0.6g, Total Carbs 11g, Net Carbs 9g, Protein 2g, Sugar 7g, Fiber 2g, Sodium 88mg, Potassium 358mg

CITRUS SALAD SAUCE

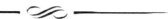

Preparation Time: 5 minutes Cooking Time: 0 minutes Serving: 4

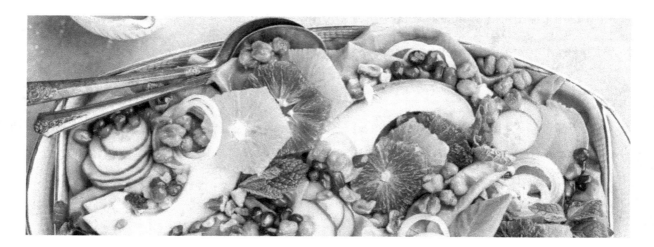

INGREDIENTS:

- 1/3 cup fresh orange juice
- 2 tbsps balsamic vinegar
- 1 tbsp extra-virgin olive oil
- salt and pepper to taste

DIRECTIONS:

Place all ingredients in a bowl.

Whisk until well-combined.

Place in a small jar and shake well before using.

Keep in the fridge for two days.

NUTRITION: Calories 43, Total Fat 4g, Saturated Fat 0.5g, Total Carbs 4g, Net Carbs 4g, Protein 0.1g, Sugar 1g, Fiber 0g, Sodium 73 mg, Potassium 103mg

ANTI-INFLAMMATORY APPLESAUCE

Preparation time: 10 minutes Cooking Time: 15 minutes Serving: 4

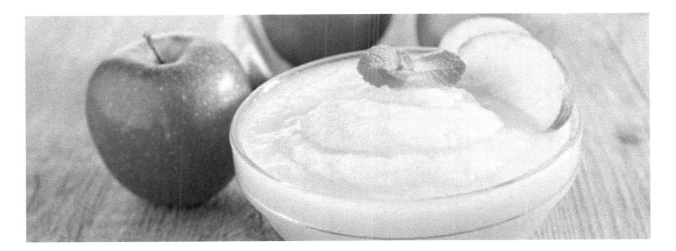

INGREDIENTS:

- 12 organic apples, peeled, cored, and sliced
- 2 tsps cinnamon
- Water for steamer pot

DIRECTIONS:

Pour water in a deep pan and place a steamer basket on top.

Place apples in the steamer and steam for 15 minutes until soft.

Place the apples in a food processor and add in cinnamon.

Pulse until smooth.

Place in containers and store in the fridge until ready to consume.

NUTRITION:

Calories 287, Total Fat 0.9g, Saturated Fat 0.1g, Total Carbs 76g, Net Carbs 62g, Protein 2g, Sugar 56 g, Fiber 14g, Sodium 6mg, Potassium 590mg

Poppy Seed-Lemon Dressing on Winter Fruit Salad

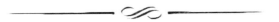

Preparation time: 10 minutes Cooking Time: 25 minutes Serving: 4

INGREDIENTS:

- 1 pear, peeled, cored and diced
- 1 apple, peeled cored and diced
- ¼ cup dried cranberries
- 1 cup cashews
- 4 oz shredded Swiss cheese
- 1 head Romaine lettuce, torn into bite size pieces
- 1 tbsp poppy seeds
- 2/3 cup vegetable oil
- ½ tsp salt
- 1 tsp Dijon-style prepared mustard
- 2 tsp diced onion
- ½ cup lemon juice
- ½ cup white sugar

DIRECTIONS:

In a blender, process salt, mustard, onion, lemon juice and sugar. Slowly pour in oil as blender is running. Continue blending until smooth and creamy. Add poppy seeds, blend one more time and set aside.

Mix well diced pear, diced apple, cranberries, cashews, Swiss cheese and lettuce in a large salad bowl.

Pour in dressing, toss well to coat.

NUTRITION: Calories 334, carbs 20g, protein 7g, fats 28g, phosphorus 172mg, potassium 409mg, sodium 177mg

JANE'S APPLE SALAD

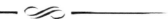

Preparation Time: 5 minutes Cooking Time: 0 minutes Serving: 4

INGREDIENTS:

- 2 cups diced apples (about 4 apples)
- ½ tsp. chopped nuts
- ½ tsp. golden grapes
- 3 Tbsps. mayonnaise
- 3 Tbsps. low-fat yogurt

DIRECTIONS:

Combine all the Ingredients.

Relax.

NUTRITION:

Calories 195kcal, Sodium 297mg, Potassium 70mg, Phosphorus 96mg, Protein 3g

Heart Healthy Chicken Salad

Preparation time: 10 minutes Cooking Time: 15 minutes Serving: 4

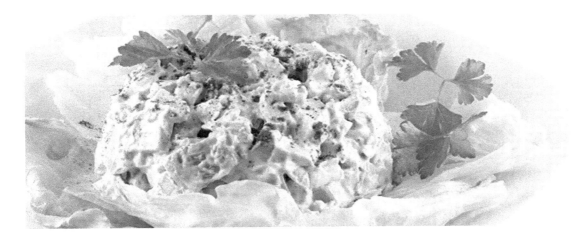

INGREDIENTS:

- 3 Tbsps. mayonnaise, low-fat
- ½ tsp. onion powder
- 1 Tbsp lemon juice
- ¼ cup celery (chopped)
- 3 ¼ cups chicken breast (cooked, cubed, and skinless)

DIRECTIONS:

Bake chicken breasts for 45 minutes at 350F. Let them cool, cut them into cubes and place them in the refrigerator.

Combine all other ingredients in a large bowl then add the chilled chicken.

Mix well and ready to serve.

Enjoy!

NUTRITION:

Calories 408, carbs 1g, protein 50g, fats 22g, phosphorus 413mg, potassium 542mg, sodium 154mg

SPINACH AND CRANBERRY SALAD

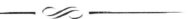

Preparation time: 10 minutes Cooking Time: 15 minutes Serving: 4

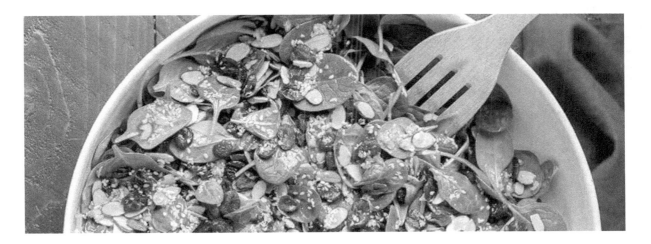

INGREDIENTS:

- ½ cup vegetable oil
- ¼ cup cider vinegar
- ¼ cup white wine vinegar
- ¼ tsp paprika
- 2 tsp. minced onion
- ½ cup white sugar
- 1 tbsp poppy seeds
- 2 tbsps toasted sesame seeds
- 1 cup dried cranberries
- 1 lb spinach, rinsed and torn into bite-size pieces
- ¾ cup almonds, blanched and slivered
- 1 tbsp butter

DIRECTIONS:

On medium heat, melt butter in a medium skillet. Add slivered almonds and toast lightly. Transfer to a plate and allow to cool.

Whisk well vegetable oil, cider vinegar, white wine vinegar, paprika, onion, sugar, poppy seeds and sesame seeds in a medium bowl.

Mix well cranberries, cooled almonds and spinach in a large salad bowl.

Pour in dressing, toss well to coat and serve.

NUTRITION:

Calories 208, carbs 15g, protein 3g, fats 19g, phosphorus 72mg, potassium 456mg, sodium 65mg

GREEN PEA SALAD

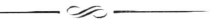

Preparation time: 10 minutes Cooking Time: 25 minutes Serving: 4

INGREDIENTS:

- 1 cup iceberg lettuce, chopped
- 2 diced celery sticks
- 1 medium green pepper, diced
- 1 red onion or chopped sweet onion
- 1 can of peas (without salt)
- 3/4 cup Mayonnaise
- 4 hardboiled eggs, sliced
- ½ tsp. grated cheese
- 2 slices of bacon or turkey bacon

DIRECTIONS:

Chop a head of lettuce and spread it at the bottom of a transparent glass container.

Pour in the celery, green pepper, onion, green peas and eggs.

Cover this layer with mayonnaise completely.

Cover with plastic wrap and refrigerate overnight.

Before serving, garnish with bacon pieces and grated cheese.

NUTRITION: Calories 264kcal, Sodium 195mg, Potassium 140mg, Phosphorus 107mg, Protein 9g

QUINOA, CILANTRO AND CRANBERRY SALAD

Preparation time: 10 minutes Cooking Time: 15 minutes Serving: 4

INGREDIENTS:

- Pepper to taste
- 1/8 tsp salt
- ½ cup dried cranberries
- ½ cup minced carrots
- ¼ cup toasted sliced almonds
- 1 lime, juiced
- ¼ cup chopped fresh cilantro
- 1 ½ tsp curry powder
- 1 small red onion, finely chopped
- ¼ cup yellow bell pepper, chopped
- ¼ cup red bell pepper, chopped
- 1 cup uncooked quinoa, rinsed
- 1 ½ cups water

DIRECTIONS:

In a saucepan, bring water to a boil and add quinoa. Cover and lower heat to a simmer and cook until water is fully absorbed, around 15-20 minutes.

Transfer quinoa into a large salad bowl and allow to cool in the fridge fully.

After an hour of cooling in the fridge, add cranberries, carrots, almonds, lime juice, cilantro, curry powder, red onion, yellow bell pepper and red bell pepper into salad bowl. Mix well.

Return bowl to the fridge and chill for another hour before serving.

NUTRITION: Calories 149, carbs 25g, protein 5g, fats 3g, phosphorus 145mg, potassium 263mg, sodium 63mg

WILD RICE SALAD

Preparation time: 10 minutes Cooking Time: 15 minutes Serving: 4

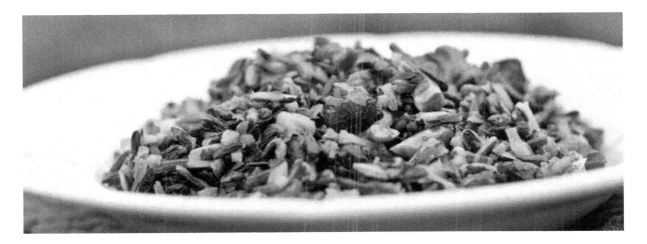

INGREDIENTS:

- 6-oz blanched slivered almonds
- 1 cup seedless red grapes
- ¼ cup diced green onion
- 2 cups cooked, cubed turkey meat
- Pepper to taste
- 1 tsp white sugar
- ¾ cup light mayo
- 1 6-oz package wild rice

DIRECTIONS:

Cook your wild rice according to package directions. Once done, allow to cool.

Whisk pepper, salt, sugar, vinegar and mayonnaise until smooth and creamy in a small bowl.

In a large salad bowl, mix grapes, onion, turkey and cooled wild rice.

Pour in the dressing and toss well to combine.

Place in the fridge for at least an hour before serving.

NUTRITION:

Calories 308, carbs 26g, protein 18g, fats 17g, phosphorus 270mg, potassium 400mg, sodium 30mg

TUNA CAPRESE SALAD

Preparation time: 10 minutes Cooking Time: 15 minutes Serving: 4

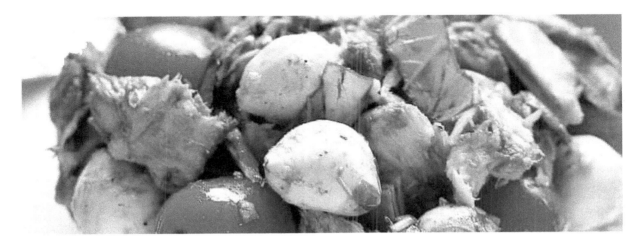

INGREDIENTS:

- 2 tsp. balsamic vinegar
- 4 tsp. extra virgin olive oil
- Pepper to taste
- 1/8 tsp salt
- 8 large fresh basil leaves
- 2 oz fresh mozzarella, sliced into ½-inch cubes
- 8 oz tomatoes, sliced thinly
- 6 oz fresh tuna steak
- 1 tsp olive oil

DIRECTIONS:

Place a large skillet with olive oil on medium heat.

Once hot, fry tuna for 3 minutes on each side. Transfer to a plate with paper towel and dab dry. Place in the fridge to cool for at least an hour.

To assemble, layer tomatoes and tuna on a plate.

Season with pepper and salt. Sprinkle with basil and mozzarella.

Drizzle balsamic vinegar and olive oil before serving.

NUTRITION:

Calories 273, carbs 9g, protein 32g, fats 13g, phosphorus 461mg, potassium 755mg, sodium 413mg

CHAPTER 4: SOUPS

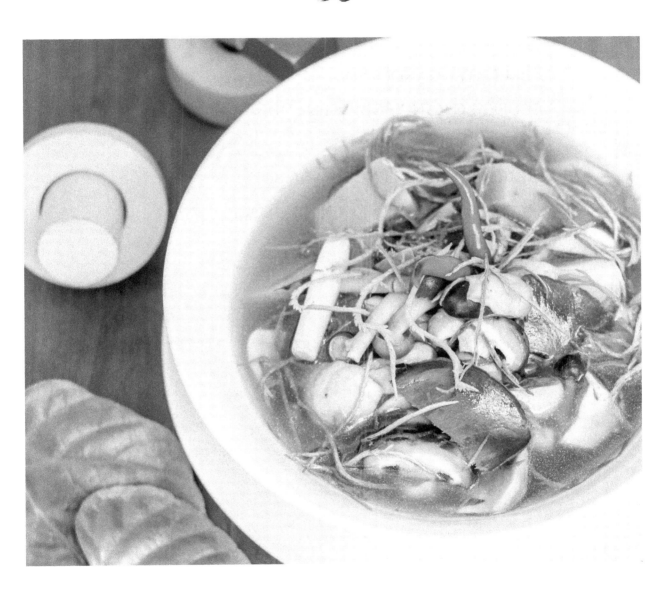

SOUPS

89. BEEF STROGANOFF SOUP

90. BUFFALO RANCH CHICKEN SOUP

91. PAPRIKA PORK SOUP

92. GREEN CHICKEN ENCHILADA SOU

93. MEDITERRANEAN VEGETABLE SOUP

94. TOFU SOUP

95. COFFEE AND WINE BEEF STEW

96. BEEF STEW

97. BACON CHEESEBURGER SOUP

Beef Stroganoff Soup

―――――――― ∽ ――――――――

Preparation time: 10 minutes Cooking Time: 30 minutes Serving: 4

INGREDIENTS:

- 2 large beef rump (sirloin) steaks (800 g/ 1.76 lbs.)
- 600 g brown or white mushrooms (1.3 lbs.)
- ¼ cup of ghee or lard (55 g/ 1.9 oz.)
- 2 cloves garlic, minced
- 1 medium white or brown onion, chopped (110 g/ 3.9 oz.)
- 5 cups bone broth or chicken stock or vegetable stock (1.2 l/ quart)
- 2 tsps of paprika
- 1 tbsp of Dijon mustard (you can make your own)
- Juice from 1 lemon (~ 4 tbsp.)
- 1½ cup sour cream or heavy whipping cream (345 g/ 12.2 oz.) - you can use paleo-friendly coconut cream
- ¼ cup freshly chopped parsley
- 1 tsp salt
- ¼ tsp freshly ground black pepper

DIRECTIONS:

Lay the steaks in the freezer in a single layer for 30 to 45 minutes. This will make it easy to slice the steaks into thin strips. Meanwhile, clean and slice the mushrooms. Fry over a medium-high heat until they're cooked through and browned from all sides. Remove the slices from the pan and place them in a bowl. Set aside for later. Do the same for the remaining slices. Grease the pan with the remaining ghee. Add in the chopped onion and minced garlic to the pan and cook until lightly browned and fragrant. Add the sliced mushrooms and cook for 3 to 4 more minutes while stirring occasionally. Then add your Dijon mustard, paprika, and pour in the bone broth. Add lemon juice and boil for 2 to 3 minutes. Add the browned beef slices and sour cream. Remove from heat. If you are using a thickener, add it to the pot and stir well. Finally, add freshly chopped parsley. Eat hot with a slice of toasted Keto Bread or let it cool down and store in the fridge for up to 5 days. Enjoy!

NUTRITION:

Calories from carbs 7%, protein 27%, fat 66%, Total carbs 10.8 g, Fiber 1.4 grams, Sugars 4.8 grams, Saturated fat 18.4 grams, Sodium 783 mg (34% RDA), Magnesium 152 mg (38% RDA), Potassium 1,398 mg (70% EMR).

Buffalo Ranch Chicken Soup

Preparation time: 20 minutes Cooking time: 30 minutes

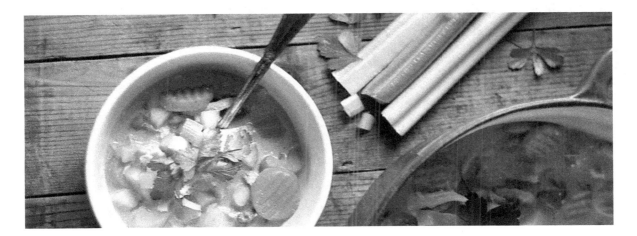

INGREDIENTS:

- 4 cups of boneless skinless chicken breast
- 2 tbsps of (I added more to mine, but made it very mild for the family)
- 4 tbsps of ranch dressing
- 2 celery stalks (chopped or sliced)
- ¼ cup of yellow onion (chopped)
- 6 tbsps of butter (salted)
- 8 ounces of cream cheese
- 1 cup of heavy whipping cream
- 8 cups of chicken broth
- 7 slices of hearty bacon

DIRECTIONS:

First, cook and shred chicken by coating the bottom of a deep-frying pan with olive oil on medium heat. Then place the chicken in a pan and cook for 5 minutes. Flip to the other side and add ¾ cup of water. Cover and cook for 7 to 10 minutes (add little drops of water occasionally). Shred after cooling. Cook and crumble bacon. I always precook bacon to make cooking a little easier. While waiting add all ingredients to a saucepan and cook on medium. When chicken and bacon are properly cooked add to the saucepan and cover. Allow to cook for 5 to 10 minutes before serving. Enjoy.

NUTRITION:

Calories: 444, Total Fat 34g, Cholesterol 133mg, Sodium 1572mg, Potassium 3mg, Carbohydrates 4g, Dietary Fiber 1g, Net Carbs 3g, Sugars 2g (all from natural sources), Protein: 28g

PAPRIKA PORK SOUP

Preparation time: 5 minutes Cooking time: 35 minutes Servings: 2

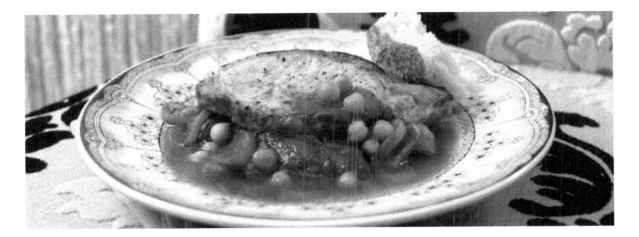

INGREDIENTS:

- 4 oz. sliced pork loin
- 1 tsp. black pepper
- 2 minced garlic cloves
- 1 cup baby spinach
- 3 cups water
- 1 tbsp. extra-virgin olive oil
- 1 chopped onion
- 1 tbsp. paprika

DIRECTIONS:

1. In a large pot, add the oil, chopped onion and minced garlic.
2. Sauté for 5 minutes on low heat.
3. Add the pork slices to the onions and cook for 7-8 minutes or until browned.
4. Stir in the spinach, reduce heat and simmer for a further 20 minutes or until pork

is thoroughly cooked through.

5. Season with pepper to serve.

NUTRITION:

Calories 165, Protein 13 g, Carbs 10 g, Fat 9 g, Sodium (Na) 269 mg, Potassium (K) 486 mg, Phosphorus 158 mg

GREEN CHICKEN ENCHILADA SOUP

Preparation time: 10 minutes Cooking time: 5 minutes Servings: 6

INGREDIENTS:

- ½ cup of salsa Verde
- 4 ounces of cream cheese, softened
- 1 cup of sharp cheddar cheese, shredded
- 2 cups of bone broth or chicken stock
- 2 cups of cooked chicken, shredded

DIRECTIONS:

Add the salsa, cream cheese, cheddar cheese and chicken stock in a blender and blend until smooth. Pour into a medium saucepan and cook on medium until hot.

NUTRITION:

Calories 346, Fat 22g, Carbohydrates 3g net, Protein 32g

Mediterranean Vegetable Soup

Preparation time: 5 minutes Cooking time: 30 minutes Servings: 4

INGREDIENTS:

- 1 tbsp. oregano
- 2 minced garlic cloves
- 1 tsp. black pepper
- 1 diced zucchini
- 1 cup diced eggplant
- 4 cups water
- 1 diced red pepper
- 1 tbsp. extra-virgin olive oil
- 1 diced red onion

PREPARATION:

Soak the vegetables in warm water prior to use.

In a large pot, add the oil, chopped onion and minced garlic.

Simmer for 5 minutes on low heat.

Add the other vegetables to the onions and cook for 7-8 minutes.

Add the stock to the pan and bring to a boil on high heat.

Stir in the herbs, reduce the heat, and simmer for a further 20 minutes or until thoroughly cooked through.

Season with pepper to serve.

NUTRITION: Calories 152, Protein 1g, Carbs 6g, Fat 3g, Sodium (Na) 3mg, Potassium (K) 229mg, Phosphorus 45mg

TOFU SOUP

Preparation time: 5 minutes Cooking time: 10 minutes Servings: 2

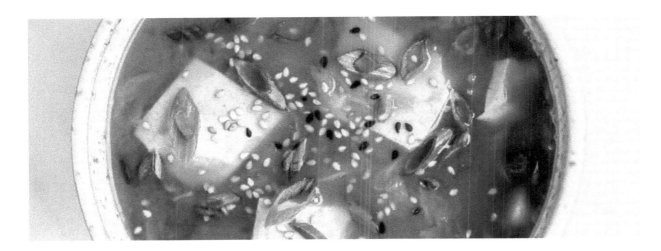

INGREDIENTS:

- 1 tbsp. miso paste
- 1/8 cup cubed soft tofu
- 1 chopped green onion
- ¼ cup sliced Shiitake mushrooms
- 3 cups Renali stock
- 1 tbsp. soy sauce

DIRECTIONS:

In a saucepan, boil the stock on high heat. Reduce heat to medium and let it simmer. Add mushrooms and cook for another 3 minutes.

Mix Soy sauce (reduced salt) and miso paste in a bowl. Add this mixture and the tofu to the stock. Simmer for nearly 5 minutes and serve with chopped green onion.

NUTRITION:

Calories 129, Fat 7.8g, Sodium (Na) 484mg, Potassium (K) 435mg, Protein 11g, Carbs 5.5g, Phosphorus 73.2mg

COFFEE AND WINE BEEF STEW

Preparation time: 20 minutes Cooking time: 3 hours 20 minutes Servings: 6

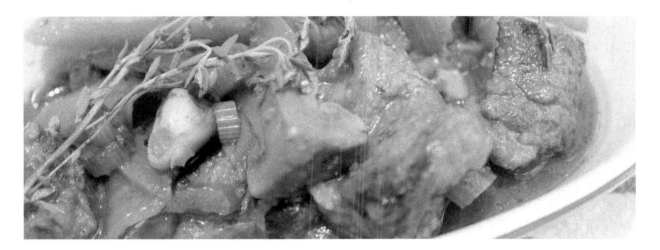

INGREDIENTS:

- Pounds Stew Meat
- 3 c. Coffee
- 1 c. Beef Stock
- 2 tbsp. Capers
- 2 tsp. Garlic
- 1 tsp. Salt
- 1 tsp. Pepper

DIRECTIONS:

Cube all stew meat and thinly slice onions and mushrooms. Heat 3 tablespoons of coconut oil in a pan. Season the beef with salt and pepper, then brown all of it in small batches. Stir mixture well. Add beef into the mixture, bring to a boil then reduce heat to low. Cover and cook for 3 hours. Serve and enjoy.

NUTRITION:

Calories 504, Fats 32.2g, Net Carbs 2.7g, Protein 42.5g

Beef Stew

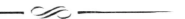

Preparation time: 10 minutes Cooking time: 1 hour Servings: 4

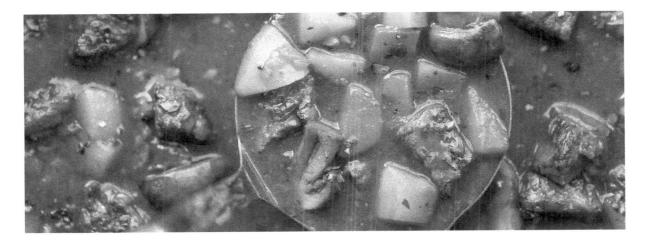

INGREDIENTS:

- 1 pound of Beef Short Rib
- 2 cups of beef broth
- 4 cloves minced garlic
- 100g onion
- 100g carrot
- 100g radishes
- ¼ tsp of Pink Himalayan Salt
- ¼ tsp of pepper
- ½ tsp of xanthan Gum
- 1 tbsp of Butter
- 1 tbsp of coconut oil

DIRECTIONS:

On medium-high heat, heat a large saucepan and add coconut oil. Then add short rib and brown on all sides. Remove from saucepan and set aside. Chop onions, carrots and radishes into bite sized pieces and mince garlic. Add onions, garlic and butter and cook for a couple of minutes. Once the onions are soft, add the broth and combine. Add the xanthan gum and mix. Allow broth mixture to come to a boil and then transfer the meat back in and cook covered for 30 minutes. Stir frequently scraping the bottom as you stir. After 30 minutes, add the carrots and radishes and cook for 30 more minutes, stirring frequently until it thickens. If you feel the need you can add more broth or some water. Serve warm and enjoy!

NUTRITION:

Calories 432.25kcal, Carbohydrates 5.5g, Protein 19.25g, Fat 36.5g, Fiber 1.5g

BACON CHEESEBURGER SOUP

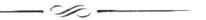

Cooking time: 40 minutes Preparation time: 20 minutes Servings: 6

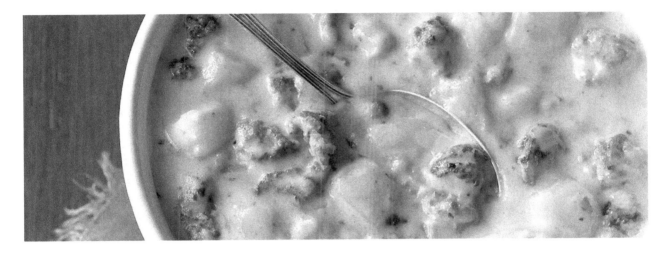

INGREDIENTS:

- 5 slices bacon
- 12 ounces of ground beef (80/20)
- 2 tbsps of butter
- 3 cups of beef broth
- ½ tsp of garlic powder
- ½ tsp of onion powder
- 2 tsps of brown mustard
- 1½ tsp of kosher salt
- ½ tsp of black pepper
- ½ tsp of red pepper flakes
- 1 tsp of cumin
- 1 tsp of chili powder
- 2½ tbsps of tomato paste
- 1 medium dill pickle, diced

- 1 cup cheddar cheese, shredded
- 3 ounces cream cheese
- ½ cup heavy cream

DIRECTIONS:

Start with cooking the bacon in a pan until crispy, then set aside. Place beef in a pot, and move it to the sides. Add butter and spices to the pan and let the spices activate for 30 to 45 seconds. Turn stove off, then finish with heavy cream and crumbled bacon. Stir well and serve. Enjoy.

NUTRITION:

_____Calories, 48.6g Fats, 3.4g Net Carbs, 23.4g Protein

CHAPTER 5:
SMOOTHIES AND OTHER DRINKS

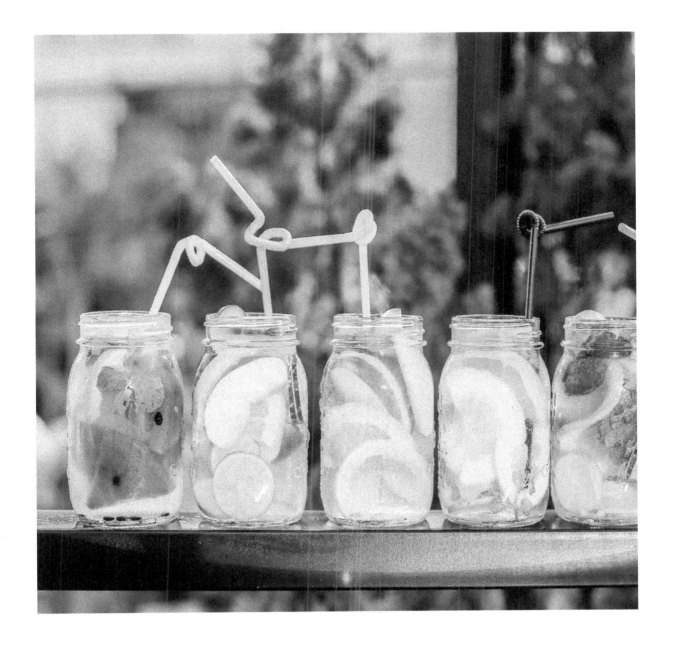

101. CINNAMON APPLE WATER

102. APPLE AND BEET JUICE MIX

103. PROTEIN CARAMEL LATTE

104. CHOCOLATE SMOOTHIE

105. LIME SPINACH SMOOTHIE

106. PROTEIN COCONUT SMOOTHIE

107. STRONG SPINACH AND HEMP SMOOTHIE

110. TOTAL ALMOND SMOOTHIE

111. ULTIMATE GREEN MIX SMOOTHIE

112. ORANGE PINEAPPLE SHAKE

113. FRUIT VANILLA SHAKE

114. PARTY PUNCH

116. ALMOND MILK

117. ROSEMARY WATERMELON WATER

119. CASHEW CREAMED COFFEE WITH COCOA NIBS

120. COCONUT CREAMED COFFEE WITH CINNAMON

121. ALMOND MILK COFFEE AND BLUEBERRY

CINNAMON APPLE WATER

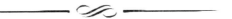

Preparation time: 5 minutes Cooking time: 5 minutes Servings: 10

INGREDIENTS:

- 1 medium apple, thinly sliced
- 10 cups water
- 2 tsp ground cinnamon
- 2 cinnamon sticks

DIRECTIONS:

Put all ingredients in a pitcher.

Refrigerate overnight.

Serve.

NUTRITION: Protein 0 g, Carbohydrates 1 g, Fat 0 g, Calories 4

APPLE AND BEET JUICE MIX

Preparation time: 5 minutes Cooking time: 5 minutes Servings: 2

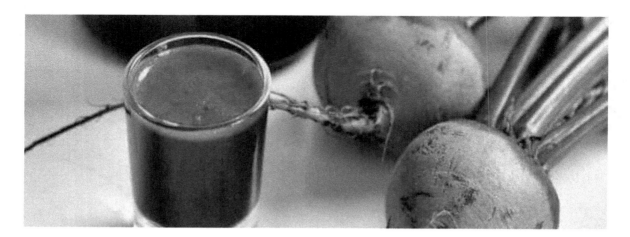

INGREDIENTS:

- ½ medium beet
- ½ medium apple
- 1 celery stalk
- 1 medium fresh carrot
- ¼ cup parsley

DIRECTIONS:

Juice all ingredients.

Pour the mixture in 2 glasses.

NUTRITION:

Protein 1g, Carbohydrates 13g, Fat 0g, Calories 53

Protein Caramel Latte

Preparation time: 4 minutes Cooking time: 6 minutes Servings: 1

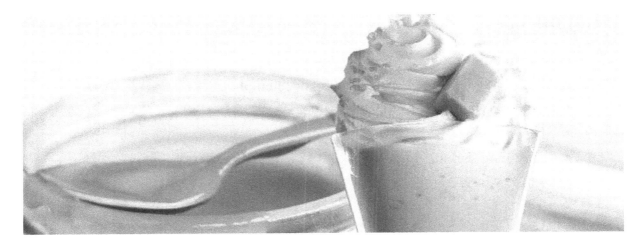

INGREDIENTS:

- ½ cup of water
- 1 scoop whey protein powder
- 2 tbsp of caramel sugar-free syrup
- 6 ounces hot coffee

DIRECTIONS:

Combine protein powder and water.

Stir in coffee and caramel syrup.

NUTRITION:

Protein 17g, Carbohydrates 1g, Fat 0g, Calories 72

CHOCOLATE SMOOTHIE

Preparation time: 5 minutes Cooking time: 5 minutes Servings: 1

INGREDIENTS:

- 1 tbsp cold water
- 1 tbsp powdered bakers cocoa, unsweetened
- 2 cups pasteurized liquid egg white
- 1 tbsp sugar
- chocolate bar shavings
- 4 tbsp whipped topping

DIRECTIONS:

Combine sugar, cold water, and cocoa.

Stir until sugar dissolves.

Add 3 tablespoons of the whipped topping and egg whites.

Top with chocolate bar shavings and 1 tablespoon whipped topping.

NUTRITION:

Protein 29g, Carbohydrates 18g, Fat 3g, Calories 215

LIME SPINACH SMOOTHIE

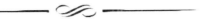

Preparation Time: 5 minutes Servings: 2

INGREDIENTS:

- 1 cup water
- 1 cup lime juice (2 limes)
- 1 green apple cored and cut into chunks
- 2 cups fresh spinach, roughly chopped
- ½ cup fresh chopped fresh mint
- ½ avocado
- Crushed ice
- ¼ tsp ground cinnamon
- 1 Tbsp natural sweetener of choice (optional)

DIRECTIONS:

Place all ingredients in your high-speed blender.

Blend for 45 - 60 seconds or until smooth and creamy.

Serve in a chilled glass.

Adjust sweetener to taste.

NUTRITION:

Calories 112, Carbohydrates 8g, Proteins 4g, Fat 10g, Fiber 5.5g

Protein Coconut Smoothie

Preparation time: 5 minutes Cooking time: 0 minutes Servings: 2

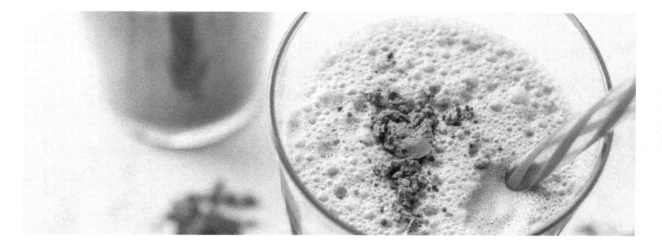

INGREDIENTS:

- 1 ½ cup coconut milk, canned
- 1 cup fresh spinach, finely chopped
- 1 scoop vanilla protein powder
- 2 Tbsp chia seeds
- 1 cup ice cubes, crushed
- 2-3 Tbsp Stevia granulated natural sweetener (optional)

DIRECTIONS:

Rinse and clean your spinach leaves from any dirt.

Place all ingredients from the list above in a blender.

Blend until you get a smoothie like consistently.

Serve in a chilled glass and it is ready to drink.

NUTRITION: Calories 377, Carbohydrates 7g, Proteins 10g, Fat 38g, Fiber 2g

STRONG SPINACH AND HEMP SMOOTHIE

Preparation time: 5 minutes Cooking time: 0 minutes Servings: 2

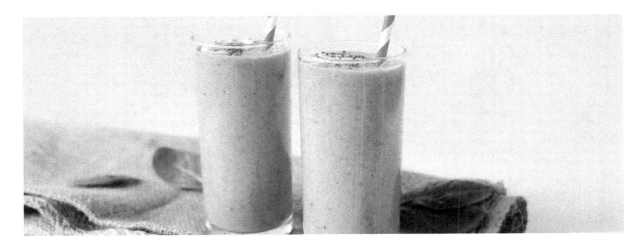

INGREDIENTS:

- 1 cup almond milk
- 1 small ripe banana
- 2 Tbsp hemp seeds
- 2 handful fresh spinach leaves
- 1 tsp pure vanilla extract
- 1 cup of water
- 2 Tbsp of natural sweetener such Stevia, Truvia...etc.

DIRECTIONS:

First, rinse and clean your spinach leaves from any dirt.

Place the spinach in a blender or food processor along with the remaining ingredients.

Blend for 45 - 60 seconds or until smooth.

Add sweetener to taste.

Serve.

NUTRITION: Calories 75, Carbohydrates 7g, Proteins 4g, Fat 6g, Fiber 3g

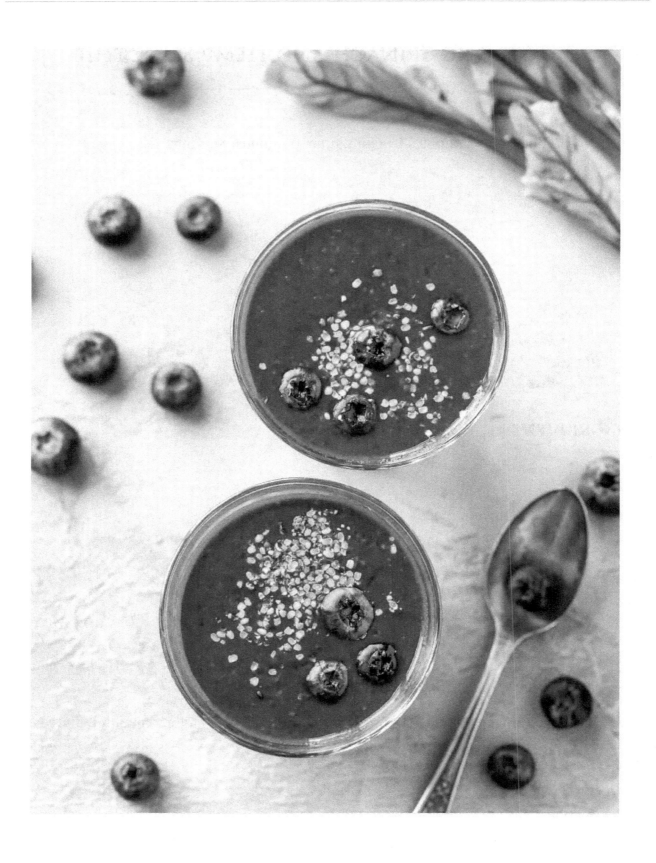

Beet Smoothie

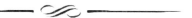

Preparation time: 10 minutes Cooking time: 0 minutes Servings: 2

INGREDIENTS:

- 10 ounces almond milk, unsweetened
- 2 beets, peeled and quartered
- ½ banana, peeled and frozen
- ½ cup cherries, pitted
- 1 tbsp almond butter

DIRECTIONS:

In your blender, mix the milk with the beets, banana, cherries and butter. Pulse well, pour into glasses and serve.

Enjoy!

NUTRITION:

Calories 165, fat 5g, fiber 6g, carbs 22g, protein 5g

TOTAL ALMOND SMOOTHIE

Preparation time: 15 minutes Cooking time: 0 minutes Servings: 2

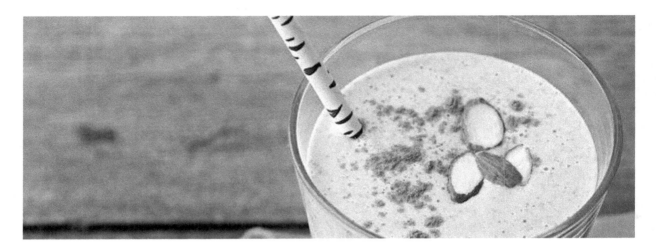

INGREDIENTS

- 1 ½ cups almond milk
- 2 Tbsp almond butter
- 2 Tbsp ground almonds
- 1 cup fresh kale leaves (or to taste)
- ½ tsp cocoa powder
- 1 Tbsp chia seeds
- ½ cup water

DIRECTIONS:

Rinse and carefully clean kale leaves from any dirt.

Add almond milk, almond butter and ground almonds in your blender; blend for 45 - 60 seconds.

Add kale leaves, cocoa powder and chia seeds; blend for another 45 seconds.

If your smoothie is too thick, pour more almond milk or water.

Serve.

NUTRITION:

Calories 228, Carbohydrates 7g, Proteins 8g, Fat 11g, Fiber 6g

Ultimate Green Mix Smoothie

Preparation time: 5 minutes Cooking time: 0 minutes Servings: 2

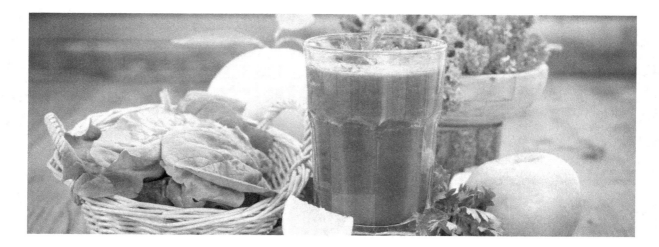

INGREDIENTS:

- Handful of spinach leaves
- Handful of collard greens
- Handful of lettuce, any kind
- 1 ½ cup of almond milk
- ½ cup of water
- ¼ cup of stevia granulated sweetener
- 1 tsp pure vanilla extract
- 1 cup crushed ice cubes (optional)

DIRECTIONS:

Rinse and carefully clean your greens from any dirt.

Place all ingredients from the list above in your blender or food processor.

Blend for 45 - 30 seconds or until smooth.

Serve with or without crushed ice.

NUTRITION:

Calories 73, Carbohydrates 4g, Proteins 5g, Fat 7g, Fiber 1g

ORANGE PINEAPPLE SHAKE

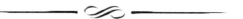

Preparation time: 3 minutes Cooking time: 5 minutes Servings: 2

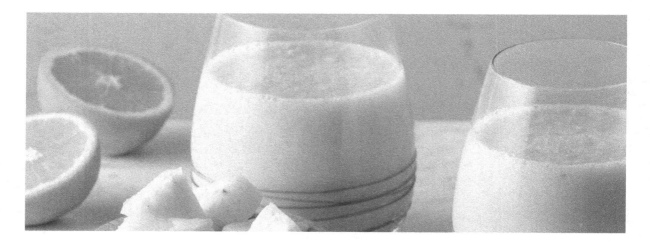

INGREDIENTS:

- ½ cup unsweetened almond milk
- ½ cup pineapple juice
- ½ cup low-cholesterol egg product
- 1 cup orange sherbet

DIRECTIONS:

Put all the ingredients in a blender. Blend for 30 seconds.

Divide into 2 servings.

Serve.

NUTRITION:

Protein 7g, Carbohydrates 36g, Fat 2g, Calories 190

VANILLA FRUIT SHAKE

Preparation time: 5 minutes Cooking time: 5 minutes Servings: 2

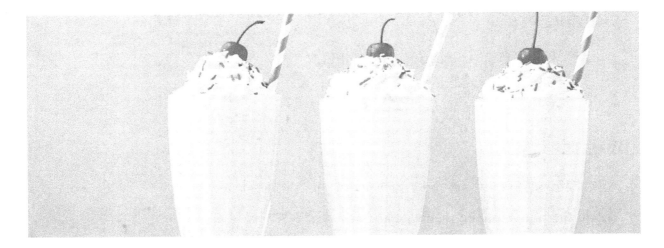

INGREDIENTS:

- 2 scoops of vanilla-flavored whey protein powder
- 8 ounces canned fruit cocktail, with juice
- 1 cup crushed ice
- 1 cup cold water

DIRECTIONS:

Mix all the ingredients in a blender.

Divide into 2 portions and serve.

NUTRITION:

Protein 23g, Carbohydrates 19g, Fat 2g, Calories 186

PARTY PUNCH

———— ❧ ————

Preparation Time: 15 minutes Cooking Time: 35 minutes Servings: 8

INGREDIENTS

- ½ cup liquid pineapple concentrate
- 1-liter of ginger ale diet
- 1 pint of lime sorbet

DIRECTIONS:

Pour the ginger ale into a large bowl or mixing bowl.

Add the pineapple concentrate and stir.

Add the sorbet with a tablespoon.

Serve when the sorbet begins to melt.

NUTRITION:

Calories 63kcal, Potassium 96mg, Sodium 26mg, Phosphorus 21mg, Protein 0g

CRANBERRY-LIME APPLE SPRITZER

Preparation Time: fifteen minutes Cooking Time: 35 minutes Servings: 8

INGREDIENTS

- 1 lime zest
- 2 sachets (12 oz) fresh or frozen blueberries
- 2/3 cup fresh lime juice (about 5 limes)
- 3 tbsp honey
- 4 cup of apple juice
- 1 bottle of cold seltzer water

DIRECTIONS:

Grate a lime to remove the lime peel (the thin and colored part of the peel), or use a vegetable peeler to strip it. Try to get just the skin, because that's where the flavor is. Juice 5 limes.

Combine blueberries, apple juice, honey and lemon zest in a large saucepan. Bring to a boil.

Lower the heat and cook until the berries burst, about 15 minutes.

Filter the mixture through a fine mesh colander and push the berries to extract as much liquid as possible.

Leave to cool to room temperature and transfer the cranberry and lime juice to a juice jar or a container with an airtight lid.

Add lime juice and shake to combine.

Store in the refrigerator.

For a spritzer, pour ¼ cup cranberry juice and lime into a tall glass and add ½ cup cold mineral water.

Add ice if desired. Add flavor to mix and shake well.

NUTRITION: Calories 36kcal, Potassium 152mg, Sodium 6mg, Phosphorus 14mg, Protein 0g

ALMOND MILK

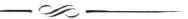

Preparation time: 5 minutes Cooking time: 15 minutes Servings: 3

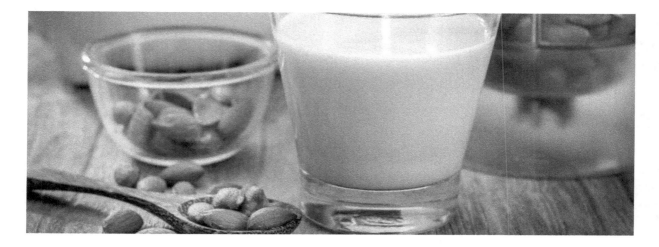

INGREDIENTS:

- 3 cups filtered water, plus water for soaking almonds
- 1 cup raw almonds
- 1 tsp vanilla extract

DIRECTIONS:

- Put raw almonds in a jar. Cover with filtered water. Cover jar and soak for 6 hours at room temperature.
- Drain the almonds. Place them in a blender.
- Add 3 cups of fresh filtered water to the blender.
- Blend for 2 minutes.
- With nut bag over the bowl, strain liquid from almond meal.
- Add vanilla extract.
- Pour almond milk into a jar. Refrigerate for 3 days.

NUTRITION:

Protein 1g, Carbohydrates 2g, Fat 3g, Calories 40

ROSEMARY WATERMELON WATER

Preparation time: 5 minutes Cooking time: 5 minutes Servings: 10

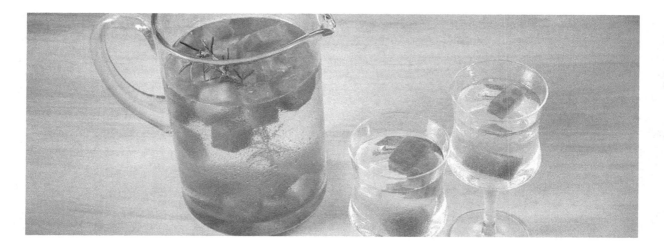

INGREDIENTS:

- 2 stems fresh rosemary
- 1 cup watermelon
- 10 cups water

DIRECTIONS:

Cut watermelon into cubes.

Put all the ingredients into a pitcher.

Refrigerate overnight before serving.

NUTRITION:

Protein 0g, Carbohydrates 1g, Fat 0g, Calories 4

ALMOND MILK CHOCOLATE COFFEE

Time: 5 Minutes Servings: 1

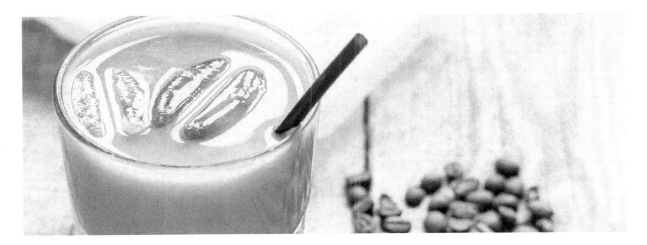

INGREDIENTS:

- 2 tsps freshly boiled water
- 1 tsp instant coffee
- 1 tsp Dutch cocoa powder
- ½ tsp green stevia, optional
- ½ cup almond milk
- ½ cup icy water

DIRECTIONS:

1. Dissolve coffee and chocolate powder in water. Pour this, along with remaining ingredients into blender; process until smooth. Pour into glass. Serve with Pecan Pancakes (Chapter 8: Snacks and Desserts).

NUTRITION:

Protein 1.2g (2% RDA), Potassium (K) 171 mg (4%), Sodium (Na) 91mg (6%)

CASHEW CREAMED COFFEE WITH COCOA NIBS

Servings: 1 Time: 5 Minutes

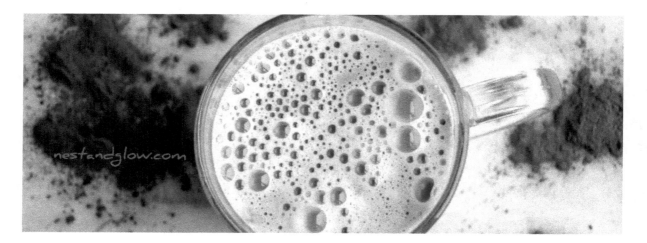

INGREDIENTS:

- 2 tsps freshly boiled water
- 1 tsp instant coffee
- ½ cup cashew milk
- ½ cup icy water
- dash nutmeg powder
- ⅛ tsp cocoa nibs, for garnish

DIRECTIONS:

1. Dissolve coffee in water. Pour this, along with remaining ingredients (except cocoa nibs) into blender; process until smooth. Pour into glass. Garnish with cocoa nibs. Serve with Oregano Pancake (Chapter 8: Snacks and Desserts).

NUTRITION:

Protein 1.51g (3%), Potassium (K) 91 mg (2%) and Sodium (Na) 7mg (0%)

Coconut Creamed Coffee with Cinnamon

Servings: 1 Time: 5 Minutes

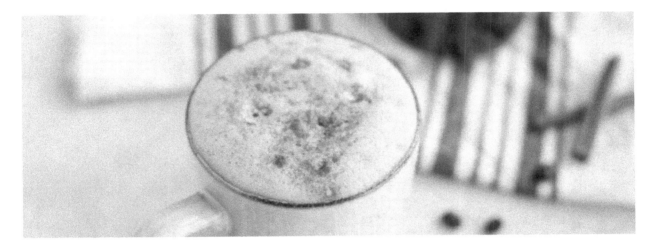

INGREDIENTS:

- 2 tsps boiled water
- 1 tsp instant coffee
- Dash of cinnamon powder
- ½ tsp green stevia, optional
- ½ cup coconut milk
- ½ cup icy water

DIRECTIONS:

1. Dissolve coffee in water. Pour this, along with remaining ingredients into blender; process until foamy. Pour into glass. Serve with Thyme Flatbread (Chapter 8: Snacks and Desserts).

NUTRITION:

Protein 2.91g (5%), Potassium (K) 355mg (8%) and Sodium (Na) 24 mg (2%)

ALMOND MILK AND BLUEBERRY COFFEE

Preparation time: 10 minutes Cooking time: 15 minutes Servings: 6

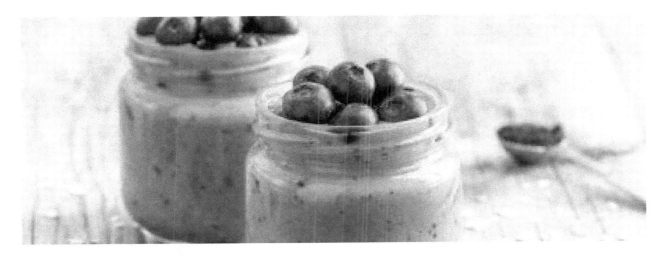

INGREDIENTS:

- 2 tsps boiled water
- 1 tsp instant coffee
- 1 tsp fresh blueberries
- ½ tsp green stevia
- ½ cup almond milk
- ½ cup icy water

DIRECTIONS:

1. Dissolve coffee in water. Pour this, along with remaining ingredients into blender; process until smooth. Pour into glass. Garnish with fresh blueberries. Serve with Basil and Almond Flour Pancakes (Chapter 8: Snacks and Desserts).

NUTRITION:

Protein 0.52g (3%), Potassium (K) 128 mg (3%) and Sodium (Na) 88mg (6%)

CHAPTER 6: LUNCH

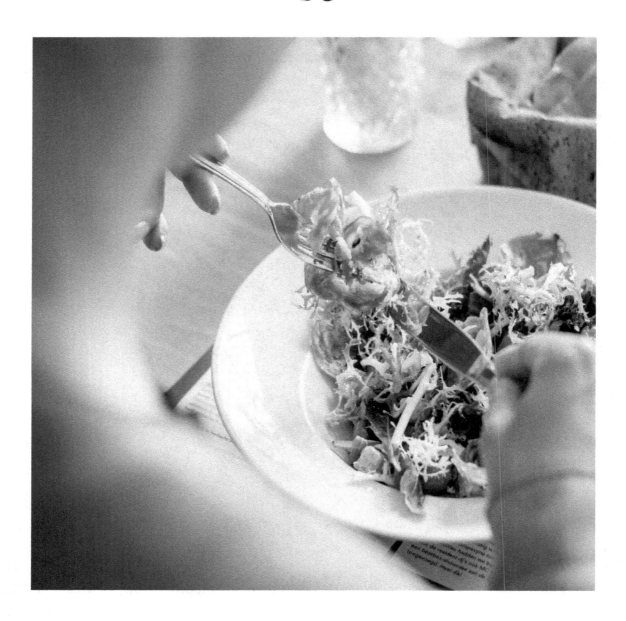

LUNCH

———— ❦ ————

SPICY AND CREAMY PORK SOUP

Preparation time: 5 minutes Cooking time: 40 minutes Servings: 3

INGREDIENTS:

- 2 tbsps olive oil
- 1 chopped shallot
- 1 chopped celery stalk
- ¾ -pound bone-in pork chops
- 1 tbsp chicken bouillon granules
- 3 cups water
- ½ tsp Tabasco sauce
- 2 pureed tomatoes
- seasoned salt and freshly cracked black pepper, to taste
- ½ tsp red pepper flakes
- 1 cup double cream
- ½ cup avocado, pitted, peeled and diced

DIRECTIONS:

Preheat a pot over a moderate-high flame and heat 1 tablespoon of oil. Cook the shallots until they are just tender.

Stir in the celery and cook until softened. Put to one side.

Heat another tablespoon of olive oil and cook the pork chops for 4 minutes until they are brown. Stir every now and then.

When the pork chops have cooled down, get rid of any bones and then cut the pork into small chunks. Put the pork and vegetables in the pot.

Add the bouillon granules, water, pureed tomatoes, red pepper flakes, salt and pepper. Partially cover the pot and simmer for 10 more minutes.

Pour in the double cream and cook until hot. Stir all the time. Drizzle Tabasco sauce on the mixture and when plated, garnish with avocado.

NUTRITION:

Calories 490, Protein 24.3g, Fat 44g,Carbs 6.1g ,Sugar 2.6g

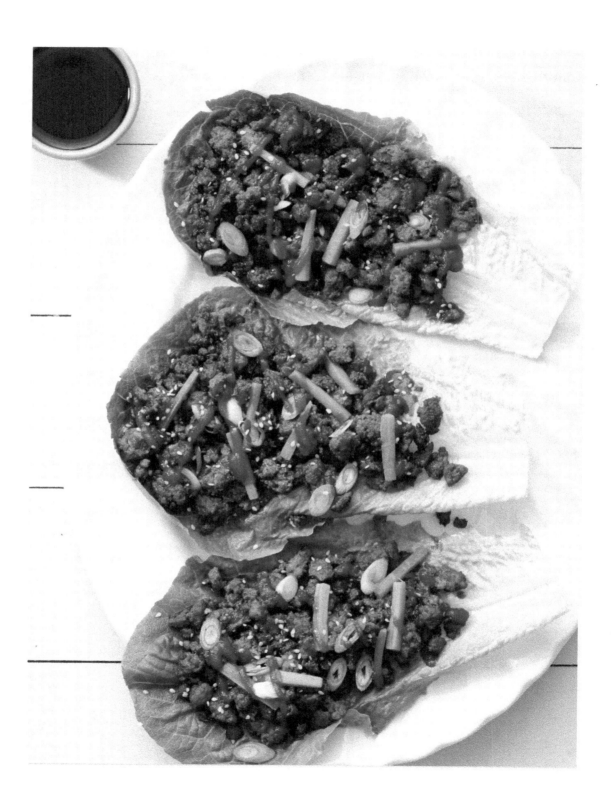

LETTUCE WRAPS WITH PORK

Preparation time: 5 minutes Cooking time: 60 minutes Servings: 3

INGREDIENTS:

- 2 tbsps apple cider vinegar
- 2 sliced spring onions
- 1 grated celery
- ¼ tsp kosher salt
- ½ -pound ground pork
- 1 deveined and finely minced jalapeno pepper
- 2 finely minced garlic cloves
- 1 ½ tsps Dijon mustard
- ½ tsp salt
- 1/3 tsp freshly cracked mixed peppercorns
- 1 tbsp Worcestershire sauce1
- 1 head lettuce
- 1 tbsp sunflower seeds

DIRECTIONS:

Whisk the vinegar together with spring onions, celery and kosher salt.

In a pan, cook the ground pork until brown, together with jalapeno pepper and garlic. This should take 7 minutes over a medium flame.

Add the Dijon mustard, salt, peppercorns and Worcestershire sauce to the pan and mix well.

Then make your wraps. Put the lettuce leaves on individual plates and divide the pork mixture among them and put the celery mixture on top. Sprinkle on sunflower seeds and roll the lettuce leaves to make wraps.

NUTRITION: Calories 125, Protein 12.5g, Fat 10.6g,Carbs 3.7g ,Sugar 1.3g

PORK STEAKS

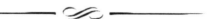

Preparation time: 5 minutes Cooking time: 40 minutes Servings: 3

INGREDIENTS:

- 4 pork butt steaks
- 2 tbsps lard at room temperature
- ¼ cup dry red wine
- ½ tsp freshly ground black pepper
- ½ tsp salt
- 1 tsp celery seeds
- ½ tsp cayenne pepper
- 1 peeled and chopped red onion
- 1 minced garlic clove

DIRECTIONS:

In a skillet that has been heated over medium heat, melt 1 tablespoon of lard. Sear the steaks for 10 minutes with the skillet covered.

Deglaze the pot with a splash of wine. Put in pepper, salt, celery seeds and cayenne pepper. Cook for 8 - 12 minutes. Put to one side.

Heat the rest of the lard and cook the garlic and onions until they are soft and fragrant. Serve with the pork butt steaks. Bon appétit!

NUTRITION:

Calories 305, Protein 22.5g, Fat 20.6g,Carbs 3.7g ,Sugar 1.3g

PORK AND VEGGIE SKEWERS

Preparation time: 5 minutes Cooking time: 30 minutes Servings: 3

INGREDIENTS:

- 2 cloves crushed garlic
- 1 tbsp Italian spice mix
- 2 tbsps fresh lime juice
- 3 tbsps tamari sauce
- 3 tbsps olive oil
- 1 ½ pounds cubed pork shoulder
- 1 thickly sliced red bell pepper
- 1 thickly sliced green bell pepper
- 1 pound small button mushrooms
- 1 onion, cut into wedges
- 1 cubed zucchini
- Wooden skewers, soaked in cold water for 30 minutes

DIRECTIONS:

First make the marinade. Combine the garlic, Italian spice mix, fresh lime juice, tamari sauce and olive oil.

Pour the marinade over the pork and marinate for 2 hours. Then thread the pork cubes, peppers, mushrooms, onions and zucchini onto skewers.

Preheat your grill and cook the skewers for about 13 minutes, turning often. Enjoy!

NUTRITION:

Calories 428, Protein 28.9g,Fat 31.6g ,Carbs 7.7g ,Sugar 4.2g

TURKEY & PUMPKIN CHILI

Preparation Time: 15 minutes Cooking Time: 41 minutes Servings: 8

INGREDIENTS:

- 2 tbsps extra-virgin olive oil
- 1 green bell pepper, seeded and chopped
- 1 small yellow onion, chopped
- 2 garlic cloves, chopped finely
- 1-pound lean ground turkey
- 1 (15-ounce) pumpkin puree
- 1 (14 ½-ounce) can diced tomatoes with liquid
- 1 tsp ground cumin
- ½ tsp ground turmeric
- ½ tsp ground cinnamon
- 1 cup water
- 1 (15-ounce) can chickpeas, rinsed and drained

DIRECTIONS:

In a big pan, heat oil on medium-low heat.

Add the bell pepper, onion and garlic and sauté approximately 5 minutes.

Add turkey and cook for about 5-6 minutes.

Add tomatoes, pumpkin, spices and water and convey to your boil on high heat.

Reduce the temperature to medium-low heat and stir in chickpeas.

Simmer covered for approximately a half-hour, stirring occasionally.

Serve hot.

NUTRITION: Calories 437, Fat 17g, Carbohydrates 29g, Fiber 16g, Protein 42g

PORK WITH BAMBOO SHOOTS AND CAULIFLOWER

Preparation time: 5 minutes Cooking time: 40 minutes Servings: 3

INGREDIENTS

- 1 ½ pounds boneless pork loin
- 1 ½ tbsps olive oil
- ½ cup vodka
- 2 tbsps oyster sauce
- ½ tsp dried marjoram
- ½ tsp garlic powder
- ¼ tsp dried thyme
- celery salt and ground black pepper to your liking
- 1 chopped yellow onion
- 1 head cauliflower florets
- 1 8-ounce can bamboo shoots

DIRECTIONS:

Put the pork loin in a bowl. Add the olive oil, vodka, oyster sauce, marjoram, garlic powder, thyme, salt and ground pepper. Combine thoroughly. Add the pork loin to a mixing dish.

In a skillet, heat 1 tablespoon of olive oil over a moderate-high heat. Sauté the onion until soft.

Put in the cauliflower florets and cook for 3 - 4 minutes until they are tender. Put this to one side.

Put another tablespoon of olive oil in the pan and heat with a high flame. Put the marinade to one side and brown the pork for 3 minutes on each side.

Put in the marinade, the cauliflower and bamboo shoots.

Cook for another 4 minutes until the sauce has thickened. Serve hot. Enjoy!

NUTRITION: Calories 356, Protein 33.1g, Fat 19.5g, Carbs 6.4g ,Sugar 3g

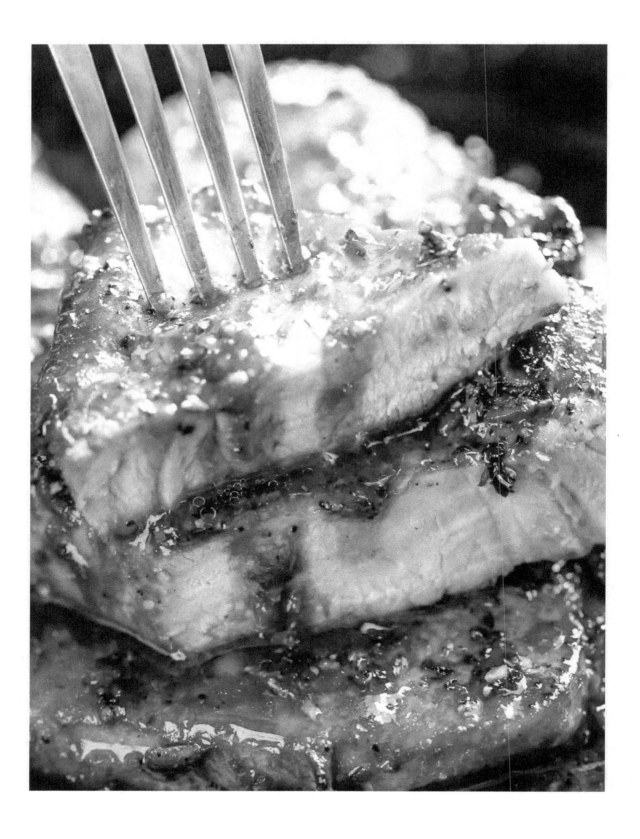

Easy Fragrant Pork Chops

———— ༖ ————

Preparation time: 5 minutes Cooking time: 20 minutes Servings: 3

INGREDIENTS:

- 2 tbsps lard, melted
- 3 minced cloves of garlic
- ½ cup thinly sliced onions
- 4 pork chops
- ½ tsp grated fresh ginger
- 4 lightly crushed allspice berries
- 2 tbsps Worcestershire sauce
- 1 tsp dried thyme
- ¼ cup dry white wine

DIRECTIONS:

Take a saucepan and melt the lard over moderate heat. Sauté the garlic and onions until they have lightly browned and are fragrant.

Add the pork to the saucepan and cook for 15 - 20 minutes, turning occasionally. Pour in the white wine, ginger, allspice berries, Worcestershire sauce and thyme.

Cook for another 8 minutes when everything should be thoroughly heated. Bon appétit!

NUTRITION:

Calories 335, Protein 18.3g, Fat 26.3g, Carbs 2.5g ,Sugar 0.8g

Slow Cooker Hungarian Goulash

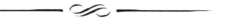

Preparation time: 5 minutes Cooking time: 20 minutes Servings: 3

INGREDIENTS:

- 1 ½ tbsps butter
- 1 pound chopped pork shoulder off the bone
- 3 crushed garlic cloves
- 1 cup chopped yellow onions
- 2 deveined and finely chopped chili peppers
- 2 ½ cups tomato puree
- 4 cups chicken stock
- 2 tsps cayenne pepper
- 1 tsp sweet Hungarian paprika
- 1 tsp ground caraway seeds
- For the Sour Cream Sauce:
- 1 cup sour cream
- 1 tsp lemon zest
- 1 bunch parsley, chopped

DIRECTIONS:

Preheat a pan over medium heat and melt the butter. Cook the pork until it has browned. Put to one side.

Sauté the garlic and onions until they are soft and aromatic.

Put the pork into the slow cooker with the onions and garlic. Add the chili peppers, tomato puree, chicken stock, cayenne pepper, paprika and caraway seeds.

Put the lid on the slow cooker and cook on a low setting for 8 10 hours.

While this is cooking, make the sour cream sauce by whisking together the sour cream, lemon zest and parsley. Serve the goulash in individual bowls topped by a spoonful of sour cream sauce. Enjoy!

NUTRITION:

Calories 517, Protein 38.2g, Fat 35.7g, Carbs 5.7, Sugar 3g

CRISPY PORK SHOULDER

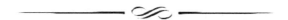

Preparation time: 5 minutes Cooking time: 40 minutes Servings: 3

INGREDIENTS:

- 1-pound pork shoulder, cut into 1-inch-thick pieces
- Salt and cayenne pepper, to taste
- 2 tbsps lard
- 2 smashed garlic cloves
- 2 sliced shallots
- 1 cup bone broth
- 2 tbsps rice vinegar
- 2 tbsps pitted and sliced Kalamata olives
- 1 tbsp fish sauce
- 1 tbsp tamarind paste
- 1 thyme sprig
- 1 rosemary sprig
- ½ cup freshly grated Asiago cheese

DIRECTIONS:

Preheat your broiler. Sprinkle the pork all over with cayenne pepper and salt.

Preheat a pan over a medium-high flame and melt the lard. Cook the garlic and shallots for 5 minutes. Put to one side.

Heat the remaining tablespoon of lard and sear the pork for 8 minutes. Turn over once and then put it to one side.

Put the rice vinegar, olives, fish sauce, tamarind paste, thyme, and rosemary in the pan and cook until the sauce reduces by half. Put in an oven dish.

Add in the pork and shallot mix and sprinkle with the Asiago cheese. Broil for about 5 minutes. Serve hot and enjoy!

NUTRITION: Calories 476, Protein 31.1g, Fat 35.3g, Carbs 6.2g, Sugar 1.2g

FRITTATA WITH SPICY SAUSAGE

———— ⤫ ————

Preparation time: 5 minutes Cooking time: 20 minutes Servings: 3

INGREDIENTS

- 3 tbsps olive oil
- 2 minced garlic cloves
- 1 cup chopped onion
- 1 tsp finely minced jalapeno pepper
- ¼ tsp cayenne pepper
- 1 tsp salt
- ½ tsp ground black pepper
- ½ pound thinly sliced pork sausage
- 8 beaten eggs
- 1 tsp crushed dried sage

DIRECTIONS:

Preheat a skillet over a moderate-high flame and heat the oil. Sauté the garlic, onion and jalapeno pepper until the onion is translucent.

Sprinkle in the cayenne pepper, salt and black pepper. Then add the sausage and cook until it has slightly browned. Stir often.

Put the mixture into a greased baking dish. Beat the eggs and pour over the sausage mixture. Scatter the dried sage on top.

Preheat the oven to 4200F and cook for 25 minutes. Bon appétit!

NUTRITION: Calories 423, Protein 22.6g, Fat 35.4g, Carbs 4.1g, Sugar 2g

PORK STIR-FRY CHINESE-STYLE WITH MUENSTER CHEESE

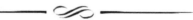

Preparation time: 5 minutes Cooking time: 40 minutes Servings: 3

INGREDIENTS:

- 1 tbsp softened lard
- 1 ½ pounds pork butt, cut into strips
- ½ tsp red pepper flakes
- celery salt and freshly ground black pepper, to taste
- 2 sliced bell peppers
- a bunch of roughly chopped scallions
- 2 tbsps Sauvignon wine
- 1 tbsp soy sauce
- ½ tsp Chinese hot sauce
- 1 tbsp peanut butter
- ¼ cup bone broth
- 3 ounces small pieces of Muenster cheese

DIRECTIONS:

Preheat a skillet over medium-high heat and melt the lard. Mix the pork strips with red pepper flakes, salt and black pepper.

Stir-fry the pork strips for around 4 minutes. Then add the bell peppers and scallions and cook for another 3 minutes.

Add the Sauvignon, soy sauce, Chinese hot sauce, peanut butter and bone broth. Stir-fry for another 2 minutes.

Put the pieces of Muenster cheese on top of this mixture and cook until the cheese melts. Bon appétit!

NUTRITION: Calories 320, Protein 39.8g, Fat 15.4g, Carbs 2.7g Sugar 1.3g

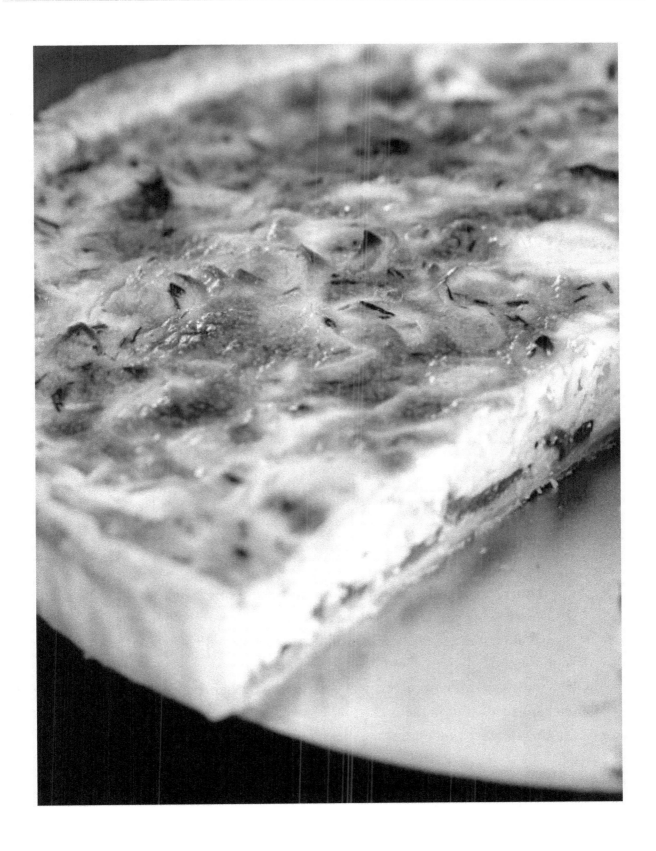

PORK AND BELL PEPPER QUICHE

Preparation time: 5 minutes Cooking time: 50 minutes Servings: 3

INGREDIENTS

- 6 lightly beaten eggs
- 1 stick melted butter
- 2 ½ cups almond flour
- 1 ¼ pounds ground pork
- Salt and pepper, to the taste
- 1 thinly sliced red bell pepper
- 1 thinly sliced green bell pepper
- 1 cup heavy cream
- ½ tsp dried dill weed
- ½ tsp mustard seeds

DIRECTIONS:

Put your oven on at 350F.

Combine an egg, butter and almond flour in a mixing bowl.

Grease a baking pan with nonstick cooking spray, roll the dough and put it in the pan.

Brown the ground pork for 3 - 5 minutes. Crumble with a spatula. Season with salt and pepper to your liking.

In a bowl, combine the other 5 eggs with the bell peppers, cream, dill weed and mustard seeds. Put in the pork.

Put this mixture in the crust and bake for 35 - 43 minutes. Eat warm and enjoy!

NUTRITION:

Calories 478, Protein 36g, Fat 4.9g, Carbs 33.5g, Sugar 1.4g

Ground Turkey with Peas & Potatoes

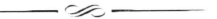

Preparation Time: 15 minutes Cooking Time: 35 minutes Servings: 8

INGREDIENTS:

- 3-4 tbsps coconut oil
- 1-pound lean ground turkey
- 1-2 fresh red chiles, chopped
- 1 onion, chopped
- Salt, to taste
- 2 minced garlic cloves
- 1 (1-inch) piece fresh ginger, grated finely
- 1 tbsp curry powder
- 1 tsp ground coriander
- 1 tsp ground cumin
- 1 tsp ground turmeric
- 2 large Yukon gold potatoes, peeled and cubed into 1-inch size
- ½ cup water
- 1 cup fresh peas, shelled
- 2-4 plum tomatoes, chopped
- ½ cup fresh cilantro, chopped

DIRECTIONS:

In a substantial pan, heat oil on medium-high heat.

Add turkey and cook for about 4-5 minutes.

Add chiles and onion and cook for about 4-5 minutes.

Add garlic and ginger and cook approximately 1-2 minutes.

Stir in spices, potatoes and water and convey to your boil

Reduce the warmth to medium-low.

Simmer covered approximately 15-twenty or so minutes.

Add peas and tomatoes and cook for about 2-3 minutes.

Serve using the garnishing of cilantro.

NUTRITION:

Calories 452, Fat 14g, Carbohydrates 24g, Fiber 13g, Protein 36g

GRILLED SALSA

Preparation time: 5 minutes Cooking time: 40 minutes Servings: 3

INGREDIENTS:

- 2 pounds of tomatillos
- 2 pounds of Roma tomatoes
- 2 large onions (cut into 3 rings)
- 6 serrano peppers
- 1 sachet of small peppers (yellow, red, orange) or large singles
- 4 large cloves of garlic
- 1 bunch of coriander leaves
- 2 tsps of salt
- 6 tbsps lemon or lime juice

DIRECTIONS:

- Cook the tomatoes and onions and grill the peppers until they are black or roasted.
- Put small amounts of each vegetable in a blender or food processor. Finely chop.
- Add the chopped garlic, cilantro, salt and lemon / lime juice and mix well.
- Cool .
- Reduce the amount of serrano peppers for a milder sauce.

NUTRITION:

Calories 33kcal, Potassium 116mg, Sodium 98mg, Phosphorus 15mg, Protein 1g

CRUNCHY CRUNCH

Preparation time: 5 minutes Cooking time: 30 minutes Servings: 3

INGREDIENTS

- 4 cup Cheerios
- 4 cup grated wheat mini
- 2 cup white diced bread
- ¼ tsp Melted margarine
- ½ tsp Oil
- ½ tsp garlic powder
- 1 tsp onion powder
- ¼ tsp black pepper

DIRECTIONS

Heat to 250F.

In a large bowl, combine the bread cubes and the cereal.

Melt the margarine in a small bowl.

Pour the margarine over the cereal mixture.

Add oil, garlic powder, onion powder and the mixture of black pepper and grains. Mix well.

Divide the mixture between 2 baking sheets.

Bake for 1 hour.

Cool and store in a covered container.

Nutrition:

Calories 191kcal, Potassium 87mg, Sodium 51mg, Phosphorus 79mg, Protein 4g

SARDINE SALAD PICKLED PEPPER BOATS

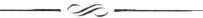

Preparation time: 5 minutes Cooking time: 40 minutes Servings: 3

INGREDIENTS

- 1 tbsp fresh parsley, chopped
- 2 (3.75-ounce) cans sardines, drained
- 2 tbsps fresh lemon
- 4 pickled peppers, slice into halves
- 1 cup scallions, chopped
- 1 tsp deli mustard
- salt and freshly ground black pepper, to taste

DIRECTIONS:

In a mixing container, thoroughly combine mustard, sardines, lemon juice, scallions, salt and black pepper.

Merge until everything is well incorporated.

Now, fill pickle boats with sardine salad. Enjoy well-chilled garnished with fresh parsley.

NUTRITION:

Calories120, Protein 12.3g, Fat 5.4g, Carbs 5.8g, Sugar 2.4g

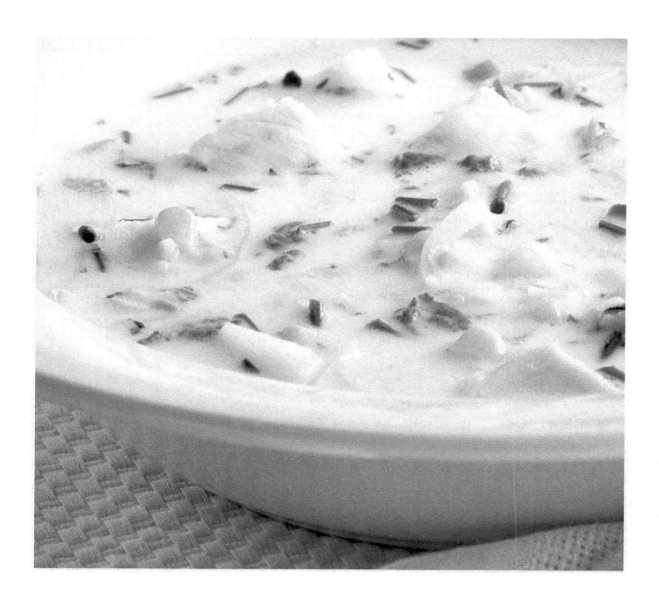

ASIAN-INSPIRED TILAPIA CHOWDER

Preparation time: 5 minutes Cooking time: 30 minutes Servings: 3

INGREDIENTS

- 1 tsp five-spice powder
- 1 celery stalk, diced
- 1 garlic clove, smashed
- ½ tsp paprika
- ¼ cup fresh mint, chopped
- ¾ cup full-fat milk
- 2 ½ cups hot water
- ½ cup scallions, sliced
- 1 bell pepper, deveined and sliced
- 3 tsps olive oil
- 1 ¼ pounds tilapia fish fillets, cut into small chunks
- 1 tbsp fish sauce

DIRECTIONS:

First off, heat olive oil in a stockpot that is preheated over a normal high heat. Heat the scallions and garlic until they are softened.

Add celery, water, fish sauce, peppers, and Five-spice powder. Put on the lid, turn the heat to medium-low and simmer for about 13 minutes longer.

Stir in fish chunks and heat an additional 12 minutes or until the fish is heated through. Include milk, stir well, and let cool.

Now, ladle into individual serving plates. Spray with paprika and serve garnished with fresh mint. Bon appétit!

NUTRITION: Calories165, Protein 25.4g, Fat 5.5g, Carbs 4g, Sugar 2.7g

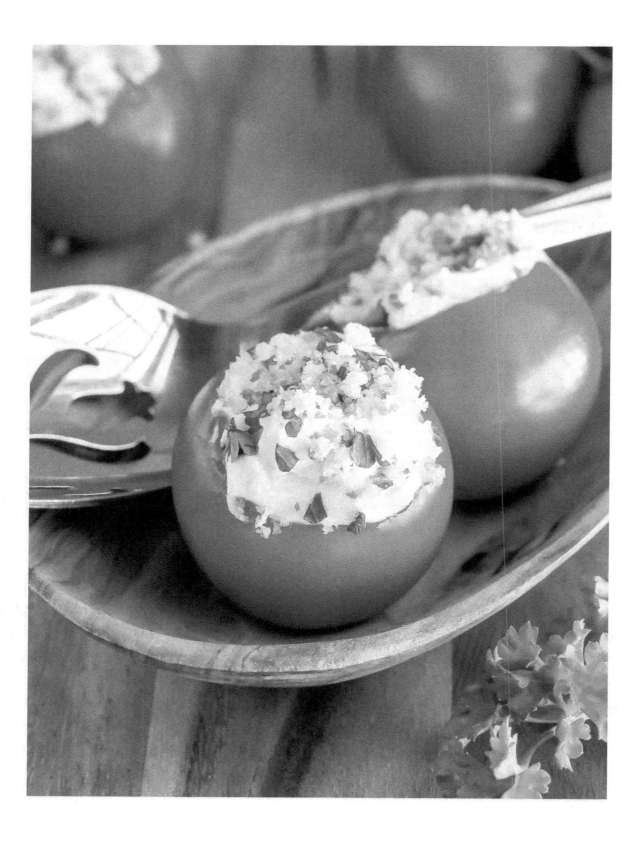

SMOKED SALMON AND CHEESE STUFFED TOMATOES

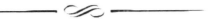

Preparation time: 5 minutes Cooking time: 20 minutes Servings: 3

INGREDIENTS:

- 2 tbsps cilantro, chopped
- ½ cup aioli
- 10 ounces smoked salmon, flaked
- 2 garlic cloves, minced
- 6 medium-sized tomatoes
- sea salt and ground black pepper, to taste
- 1 tsp yellow mustard
- 1 red onion, finely chopped
- 1 tbsp white vinegar
- 1 ½ cups Monterey Jack cheese, shredded

DIRECTIONS:

Preheat an oven to 400F.

In a mixing container, thoroughly mix the garlic, salmon, onion, cilantro, aioli, mustard, vinegar, salt and pepper.

Cut your tomatoes in half horizontally; then, scoop out pulp and seeds.

Now, stuff tomatoes with the filling and bake until they are thoroughly heated or cooked, and the tops are golden, for about 20 minutes.

Include the shredded cheese and put it in the oven for a further 5 minutes. Bon appétit!

NUTRITION:

Calories303, Protein 17g, Fat 22.9g, Carbs 6.8g, Sugar 2.2g

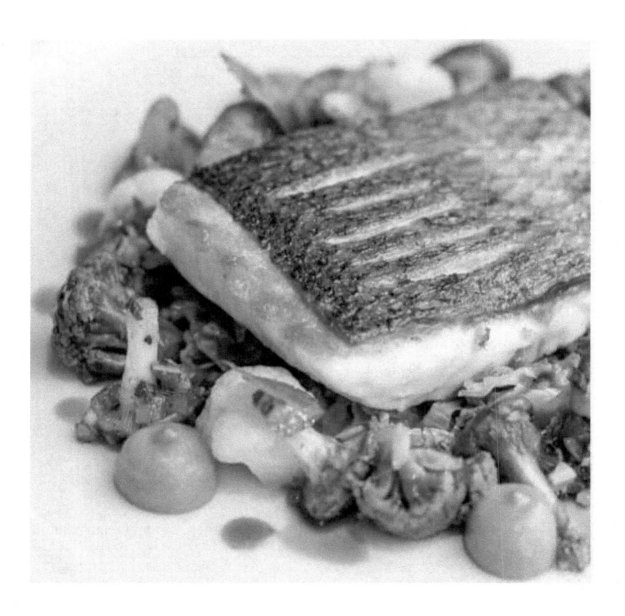

CHILEAN SEA BASS WITH CAULIFLOWER AND CHUTNEY

Preparation time: 5 minutes Cooking time: 40 minutes Servings: 3

INGREDIENTS

- 1 ½ pounds wild Chilean sea bass
- 1 onion, thinly sliced
- Sea salt and freshly ground black pepper, to taste
- 2 bell peppers, thinly sliced
- 1-pound cauliflower, cut into florets
- 1 tsp cayenne pepper
- 2 tbsps olive oil, for drizzling
- For Tomato Chutney:
- 2 garlic cloves, sliced
- 1 tsp olive oil
- 1 cup ripe on-the-vine plum tomatoes
- ¼ tsp black pepper
- ½ tsp kosher salt

DIRECTIONS:

Heat 1 tbsp of olive oil in a pan that is preheated over a normal flame.

Now, heat the bell peppers, cauliflower florets, and onion until they are slightly tender; then, season with black pepper, salt and cayenne pepper; set aside.

Now, preheat another tablespoon of olive oil. Sear sea bass on each side for about 5 minutes.

To make chutney, heat 1 teaspoon of olive oil in a pan over a normal high heat. Sauté the garlic until just browned and also aromatic.

Include the plum tomatoes and cook, occasionally stirring, until heated through, or for about 10 minutes. Season with salt and pepper.

Share seared fish among 4 serving plates. Serve garnished with sautéed cauliflower mixture and tomato chutney. Enjoy!

NUTRITION:

Calories 291, Protein 42.5g, Fat 9.5g, Carbs 3.5g, Sugar 1.4g

GROUND TURKEY WITH VEGGIES

———— ∽ ————

Preparation Time: 15 minutes Cooking Time: 12 minutes Servings: 4

INGREDIENTS:

- 1 tbsp sesame oil
- 1 tbsp coconut oil
- 1-pound lean ground turkey
- 2 tbsps fresh ginger, minced
- 2 minced garlic cloves
- 1 (16-ounce) bag vegetable mix (broccoli, carrot, cabbage, kale and Brussels sprouts)
- ¼ cup coconut aminos
- 2 tbsps balsamic vinegar

DIRECTIONS:

In a big skillet heat both oils on medium-high heat.

Add turkey, ginger and garlic and cook approximately 5-6 minutes.

Add vegetable mix and cook approximately 4-5 minutes.

Stir in coconut aminos and vinegar and cook for about 1 minute.

Serve hot.

NUTRITION:

Calories 234, Fat 9g, Carbohydrates 9g, Fiber 3g, Protein 29g

Ground Turkey with Asparagus

Preparation Time: 15 minutes Cooking Time: fifteen minutes Servings: 8

INGREDIENTS:

- 1¾ pound lean ground turkey
- 2 tbsps sesame oil
- 1 medium onion, chopped
- 1 cup celery, chopped
- 6 garlic cloves, minced
- 2 cups asparagus, trimmed and cut into 1-inch pieces
- 1/3 cup coconut aminos
- 2½ tsps ginger powder
- 2 tbsps organic coconut crystals
- 1 tbsp arrowroot starch
- 1 tbsp cold water
- ¼ tsp red pepper flakes, crushed

DIRECTIONS:

Heat a substantial nonstick skillet on medium-high heat.

Add turkey and cook for approximately 5-7 minutes or till browned.

With a slotted spoon transfer the turkey inside a bowl and discard the grease from skillet.

In exactly the same skillet, heat oil on medium heat.

Add onion, celery and garlic and sauté for about 5 minutes.

Add asparagus and cooked turkey minimizing the temperature to medium-low.

Meanwhile inside a pan mix together coconut aminos, ginger powder and coconut crystals n medium heat and convey to some boil.

In a smaller bowl, mix together arrowroot starch and water.

Slowly, add arrowroot mixture, stirring continuously.

Cook approximately 2-3 minutes.

Add the sauce in s killed with turkey mixture and stir to blend.

Stir in red pepper flakes and cook for approximately 2-3 minutes.

Serve hot.

NUTRITION:

Calories: 309, Fat 20g, Carbohydrates 19g, Fiber 2g, Protein 28g

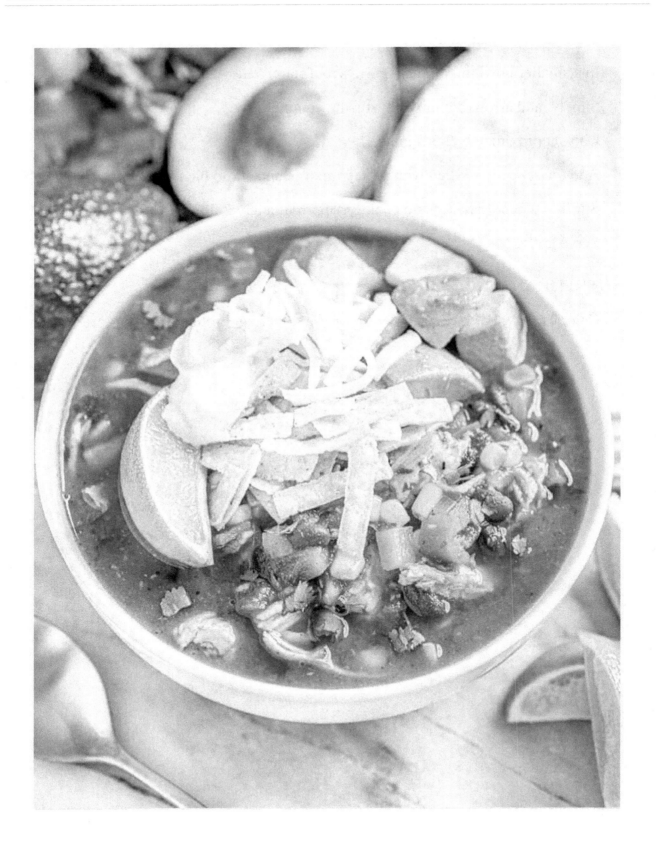

CHICKEN TORTILLA SOUP

Preparation Time: 5 minutes Cooking Time: 35 minutes Servings: 8

INGREDIENTS

- 1 medium onion, finely chopped
- 3 garlic cloves, minced
- 1 tbsp olive oil
- 2 tsps of chili powder
- 1 tsp oregano or Italian herbs
- 2 fresh tomatoes, chopped
- 1 10 oz. may be low in sodium
- chicken soup
- 1 10-oz. can water
- 1 cup corn
- 1 Ground corn
- 1 4 oz. chopped green peppers
- ¼ tsp chopped cilantro
- 3 boiled and cut chicken fillets
- lemon juice to taste
- cumin to taste
- green onions, finely chopped for garnish

DIRECTIONS:

Fry the onion and garlic in the oil.

Add the chicken, chili powder, oregano (or Italian herbs), chicken broth, water, corn, corn, cilantro and peppers and cook over medium heat for 30 minutes.

You can add lemon juice and cumin to taste.

NUTRITION: Calories 148kcal, Potassium 285mg, Sodium 142mg, Phosphorus 64mg,

Protein 16g

CHAPTER 7: DINNER

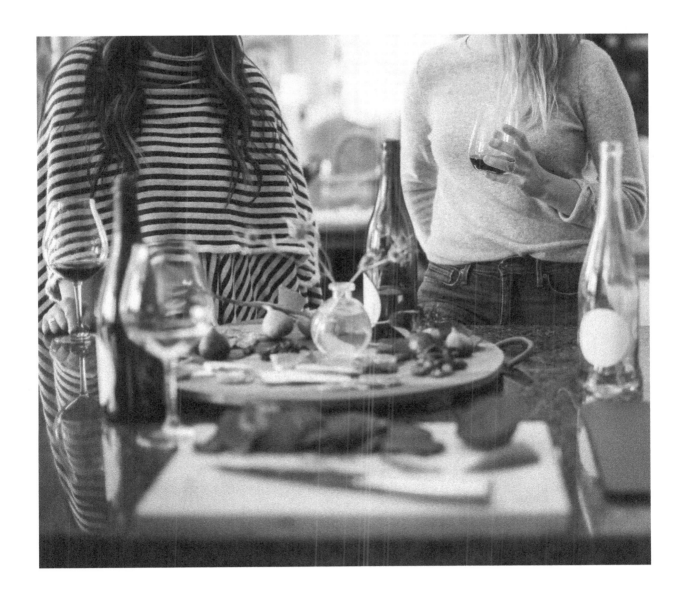

DINNER

DINNER

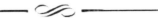

SHRIMP AND ZUCCHINI SKEWERS

Preparation Time: 5 Minutes Cooking Time: 20 minutes Servings: 4

INGREDIENTS:

- Zucchini
- Prawns
- Cold water

DIRECTIONS:

As simple as alternating slices of zucchini rolled with prawns in the middle and roasting on a griddle a couple of minutes per side. Squeeze the zucchini slices a little first and then pass them through cold water, so that they do not break when rolled.

NUTRITION:

Calories 87, Calories from Fat (13 % RDA), Total Fat 2g (2%), Saturated Fat 1g (2%), Monounsaturated Fat 0g, Polyunsaturated Fat 0g, Cholesterol 0mg, Sodium 30mg (1%), Total Carbohydrates 17g (6%), Dietary Fiber 5g (22%), Sugars 13g, Protein 7g

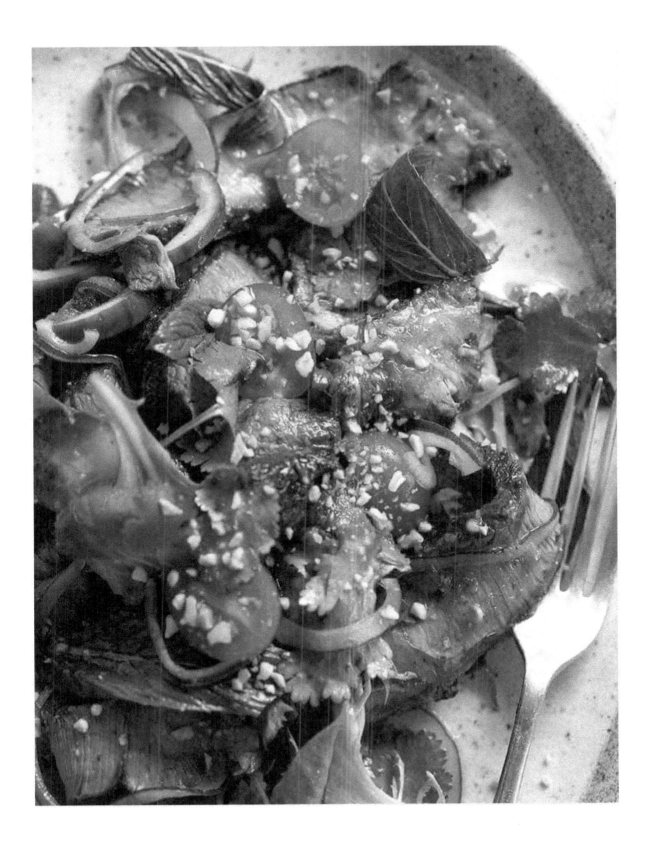

THAI STEAK SALAD WITH HERBS AND ONIONS

Preparation Time: 5 Minutes Cooking Time: 30 minutes Servings: 4

INGREDIENTS:

- 1 flank or rump steak (600 g)
- Salt
- 1 tbsp peanut oil
- Two red onions
- 1 piece Ginger (20 g)
- 1 red chili pepper
- 1 cucumber
- 3 handful Asian herbs (30 g)
- 1 tbsp rice vinegar
- 3 tbsps lime juice
- 2 tbsps fish sauce
- 1 tsp honey
- Paprika
- Chili powder
- Pepper
- meat

DIRECTIONS:

Rinse meat, one flank or rump steak, pat dry and salt. Heat the peanut oil and then fry the steak on both sides for 6-8 minutes over high heat. Remove meat from the frying pan and let it rest.

Meanwhile, peel onions and ginger. Halve onions and cut into strips. Chop ginger. Cut chili pepper into half lengthwise remove seeds, wash and cut into fine rings. Clean the cucumber, wash, quarter it and slice it. Wash Asian herbs, shake dry and peel off leaves.

Add ginger with vinegar, lime juice, fish sauce, honey and 2-3 tablespoons water to a dressing, season with paprika, chili powder, salt, and pepper.

Slice the meat and arrange with herbs, chili rings, cucumber and onions on a plate and drizzle with the dressing.

NUTRITION:

Calories: 390 kcal

CUCUMBER ROLLS ON CAULIFLOWER SALAD

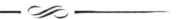

Preparation Time: 5 Minutes Cooking Time: 30 minutes Servings: 4

INGREDIENTS:

- Two small cucumbers (600 g)
- 1 carrot
- ½ orange pepper
- 1 pole celery
- 1 avocado
- 2 tbsps sprouts
- salt
- pepper
- 1 cauliflower
- 50 g raisins
- 3 tbsps. Olive oil
- 3 tbsps. lemon juice
- 1 msp. Ground cumin (knife tip)
- One pinch cinnamon
- Chili flakes
- 4 stems parsley

DIRECTIONS:

Clean cucumbers wash them and slice or slice lengthwise into skinny slices; cut the slices of cucumber into narrow, long strips.

Peel carrot. Halve, corer and wash the pepper. Clean and wipe the celery stick. Cut everything into thin finger-length strips.

Halve the avocado, remove the core, remove the pulp from the skin and cut into small slices. Wash and rinse sprouts thoroughly. Bundle some vegetable strips and wrap with a few shots in 1 slice of cucumber, season with salt and pepper. Keep cold until serving.

Clean cauliflower, wash and divide into small florets. Prepare the cauliflower in boiling salted water for about 5 minutes. Then drain, quench and let cool. Finely chop cauliflower, mix with raisins and oil. Season the cabbage with lemon juice, salt, pepper, cumin, cinnamon and chili flakes.

Wash parsley shake dry and chop leaves. Spread cauliflower on a plate. Add 2-3 cucumber rolls and parsley.

NUTRITION:

Calories: 246 kcal

STUFFED ZUCCHINI BOATS WITH GOAT CHEESE

Preparation Time: 15 minutes Cooking time: 30 minutes Servings: 4

INGREDIENTS:

- 1 cup ground chicken
- 3 oz goat cheese, crumbled
- 2 zucchinis, trimmed
- 1 tbsp sour cream
- ½ tsp salt
- ½ tsp chili flakes
- ½ tsp dried oregano
- 1 tbsp tomato sauce
- 4 tsps butter

DIRECTIONS:

Cut zucchini into lengthwise boards.

Scoop the zucchini meat.

Then mix up together ground chicken, goat cheese, salt, chili flakes, dried oregano, and fill the zucchini boats.

Then top them with sour cream and butter.

Wrap zucchini boats in the foil and transfer in the preheated to the 360F oven.

Bake zucchini for 30 minutes.

Then discard the foil and transfer cooked zucchini boats in the serving plates.

NUTRITION: calories 220, fat 14.8, fiber 1.2, carbs 4.2, protein 18

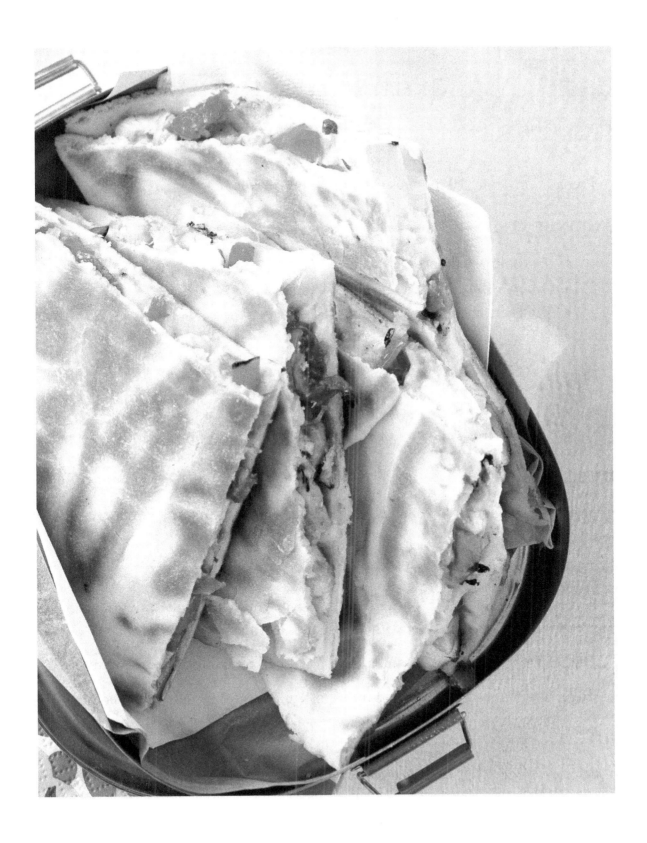

GREEK STYLE QUESADILLAS

Preparation Time: 10 minutes Cooking time: 10 minutes Servings: 4

INGREDIENTS:

- 4 whole wheat tortillas
- 1 cup Mozzarella cheese, shredded
- 1 cup fresh spinach, chopped
- 2 tbsp Greek yogurt
- 1 egg, beaten
- ¼ cup green olives, sliced
- 1 tbsp olive oil
- 1/3 cup fresh cilantro, chopped

DIRECTIONS:

In the bowl, combine together Mozzarella cheese, spinach, yogurt, egg, olives, and cilantro.

Then pour olive oil in the skillet.

Place one tortilla in the skillet and spread it with Mozzarella mixture. Top it with the second tortilla and spread it with cheese mixture again.

Then place the third tortilla and spread it with all remaining cheese mixture.

Cover it with the last tortilla and fry it for 5 minutes from each side over the medium heat.

NUTRITION:

calories 193, fat 7.7, fiber 3.2, carbs 23.6, protein 8.3

EASY PARMESAN CRUSTED TILAPIA

Preparation time: 5 minutes Cooking time: 30 minutes Servings: 3

INGREDIENTS

- ¾ cup grated Parmesan cheese
- 1/3 tsp salt
- ¼ tsp red pepper flakes, crushed
- 1-pound tilapia fillets, cut into 4
- 1/3 tsp ground black pepper
- 2 tbsps olive oil

DIRECTIONS:

Start with seasoning the fish fillets with salt, black pepper and red pepper flakes.

Now, brush tilapia fillets with olive oil; press them into the Parmesan cheese.

Put fish fillets on a foil-lined baking sheet. Bake for approximately 10 minutes or until fish fillets is opaque.

NUTRITION:

Calories 222, Protein 27.9g, Fat 12.6g, Carbs 0.9g, Sugar 0g

CREAMY PENNE

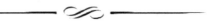

Preparation Time: 10 minutes Cooking time: 25 minutes Servings: 4

INGREDIENTS:

- ½ cup penne, dried
- 9 oz chicken fillet
- 1 tsp Italian seasoning
- 1 tbsp olive oil
- 1 tomato, chopped
- 1 cup heavy cream
- 1 tbsp fresh basil, chopped
- ½ tsp salt
- 2 oz Parmesan, grated
- 1 cup water, for cooking

DIRECTIONS:

Pour water in the pan, add penne, and boil it for 15 minutes. Then drain water.

Pour olive oil in the skillet and heat it up.

Slice the chicken fillet and put it in the hot oil.

Sprinkle chicken with Italian seasoning and roast for 2 minutes from each side.

Then add fresh basil, salt, tomato, and grated cheese.

Stir well.

Add heavy cream and cooked penne.

Cook the meal for 5 minutes more over the medium heat. Stir it from time to time.

NUTRITION: calories 388, fat 23.4g, fiber 0.2g, carbs 17.6g, protein 17.6g

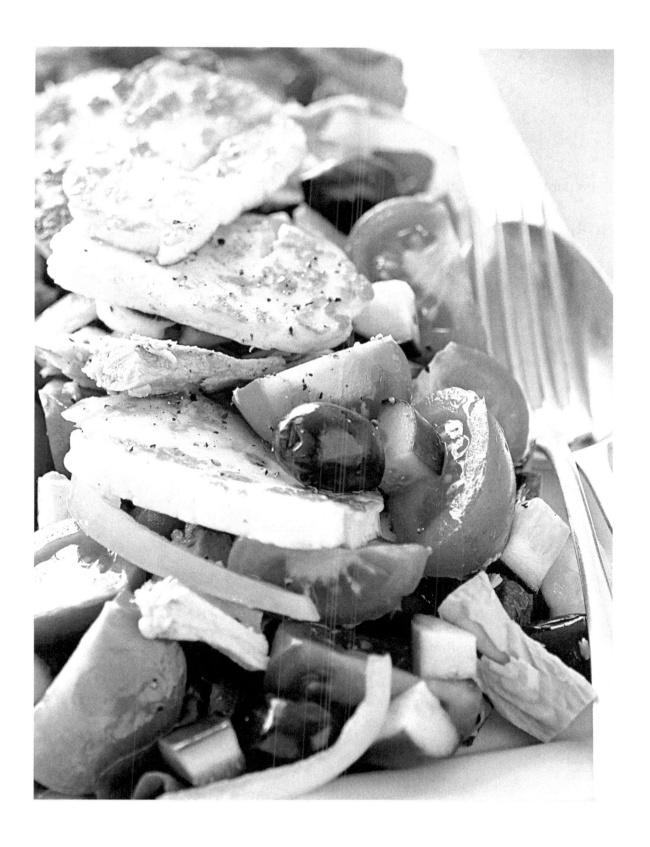

GRILLED HALLOUMI AND TUNA SALAD

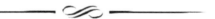

Preparation time: 5 minutes Cooking time: 20 minutes Servings: 3

INGREDIENTS:

- ½ cup radishes, thinly sliced
- 1 cup halloumi cheese, cubed
- 2 cucumbers, thinly sliced
- 2 tbsps sunflower seeds
- 1 red onion, thinly sliced
- ½ head Romaine lettuce
- 1 ½ tbsps extra-virgin olive oil
- Sea salt and black pepper, to taste
- Dried rosemary, to taste
- 1 can light tuna fish in water, rinsed
- 2 medium-sized Roma tomatoes, sliced
- 1 tbsp lime juice

DIRECTIONS:

Grill halloumi cheese over normal high heat.

Now, toss grilled halloumi cheese with the remaining ingredients. Bon appétit!

NUTRITION:

Calories 199, Protein 14.2g, Fat 10.6g, Carbs 6.1g, Sugar 4.2g

Colorful Tuna Salad with Bocconcini

———— ✀ ————

Preparation time: 5 minutes Cooking time: 40 minutes Servings: 3

INGREDIENTS:

- 1 green bell pepper, sliced
- 2 cans tuna in brine, drained
- ¼ tsp black peppercorns, preferably freshly ground
- 1 tbsp oyster sauce
- 1 head iceberg lettuce
- 1 tsp Pasilla chili pepper, finely chopped
- 2 garlic cloves, minced
- 2 tsps peanut butter
- ½ cup radishes, sliced
- 1 yellow bell pepper, sliced
- ½ cup Kalamata olives, pitted and sliced
- ½ cup yellow onion, thinly sliced
- 1 tsp olive oil
- 8 ounces bocconcini
- 1 cucumber, sliced
- 1 tomato, diced
- 1 tsp champagne vinegar

DIRECTIONS:

Mix cucumbers, iceberg lettuce, peppers, onion, tuna, radishes, tomatoes and Kalamata olives in a salad container.

In a small mixing dish, thoroughly mix champagne vinegar, olive oil, peanut butter, oyster sauce black peppercorns, and garlic.

Include this vinaigrette to the salad bowl; ensure to toss until everything is well coated.

Now, top with bocconcini and serve well-chilled. Bon appétit!

NUTRITION:

Calories 273, Protein 34.2g, Fat 11.7g, Carbs 6.7g, Sugar 2.5g

TUNA FILLETS WITH GREENS

———————— ⌒⌒ ————————

Preparation time: 5 minutes Cooking time: 10 minutes Servings: 3

INGREDIENTS

- 3 tbsps olive oil, plus more for drizzling
- 1 fresh lime, sliced
- 6 tuna fillets
- Salt and ground black pepper, to your liking
- 2 tsps yellow mustard
- 2 cups baby spinach
- 1 yellow onion, thinly sliced
- 1 tbsps apple cider vinegar
- Salt and red pepper flakes, to taste
- 1 cup rocket lettuce
- ½ cup radishes, thinly sliced

DIRECTIONS:

Begin by preheating your oven to 450F. Now, coat a baking dish with parchment paper or a Silpat mat.

Drizzle each tuna fillet with olive oil; season with pepper and salt.

Transfer tuna fillets to the baking dish. Top with lime slices and bake 8 to 12 minutes.

In a mixing container, whisk the vinegar, salt, mustard and red pepper flakes.

Distribute baby spinach, onion rocket lettuce, and radishes on 6 serving plates. Now, drizzle with vinegar/mustard mixture. Finally, top with tuna fillets. Bon appétit!

NUTRITION: Calories 444, Protein 21.9g, Fat 38.2g, Carbs 4.7g, Sugar 1.5g

Coconut Chicken Curry

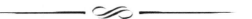

Preparation time: 10 minutes Cooking Time: 40 minutes Servings: 6

INGREDIENTS:

- 1 small sweet onion
- 2 tsps minced garlic
- 1 tsp grated ginger
- 3 tbsps olive oil
- 6 boneless, skinless chicken thighs
- 1 tbsp curry powder
- ¾ cup of water
- ¼ cup of coconut milk
- 2 tbsps cilantro, chopped

DIRECTIONS:

Place a medium saucepan or skillet on medium heat, add 2 tablespoons oil.

Add chicken and stir-cook until evenly brown, about 8-10 minutes. Set aside.

Add remaining oil. Add onion, ginger, garlic, and stir-cook until softened, about 3-4 minutes.

Mix in curry powder, water and coconut milk. Add chicken, stir the mixture and boil it.

Cover and simmer the mixture over low heat for another 25 minutes until chicken is tender.

Serve warm with cilantro on top.

NUTRITION: Calories 258, Fat 13g, Phosphorus 151mg, Potassium 242mg, Sodium 86mg, Carbohydrates 2g, Protein 25g

ONE-POT SEAFOOD STEW

Preparation time: 5 minutes Cooking time: 20 minutes Servings: 3

INGREDIENTS

- 2 garlic cloves, pressed
- ½ pound shrimp
- 1 tsp Italian seasonings
- 1 celery stalk, chopped
- 1 cup hot water
- 2 tomatoes, pureed
- 2 tbsps dry white wine
- ½ tsp lemon zest
- ½ pound mussels
- 1 tsp saffron threads
- Salt and ground black pepper, to taste
- ½ stick butter, at room temperature
- 2 cups shellfish stock
- 2 onions, chopped

DIRECTIONS:

Dissolve the butter in a stockpot over a normal heat. Heat the onion and garlic until aromatic.

After that, stir in pureed tomatoes; cook for about 8 minutes or until heated through.

Include the remaining ingredients and bring to a rapid boil. Decrease the heat to a simmer and heat an additional 4 minutes.

Ladle into individual bowls and enjoy warm.

NUTRITION: Calories209, Protein 15.2g, Fat 12.6g, Carbs 6.6g, Sugar 3.1g

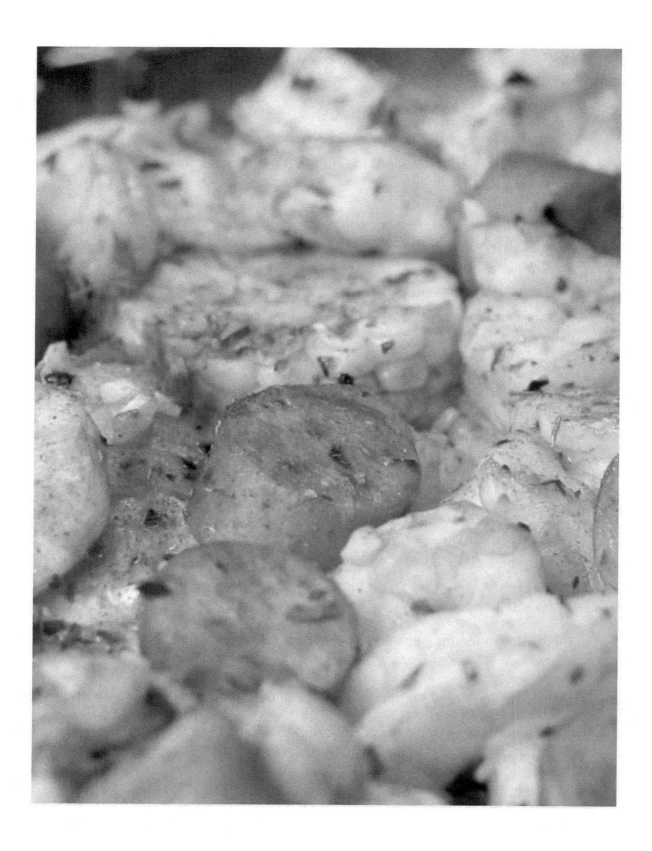

SEAFOOD AND ANDOUILLE MEDLEY

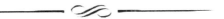

Preparation time: 5 minutes Cooking time: 40 minutes Servings: 3

INGREDIENTS:

- 2 andouille sausages, cut crosswise into ½ -inch-thick slices
- ½ stick butter, melted
- 2 tomatoes, pureed
- 2 tbsps fresh cilantro, chopped
- ½ pound skinned sole, cut into chunks
- 1/3 cup dry white wine
- 1 shallot, chopped
- 2 garlic cloves, finely minced
- 1 tbsp oyster sauce
- 3/4 cup clam juice
- 20 sea scallops

DIRECTIONS:

Dissolve the butter in a heavy-bottomed pot over medium-high heat. Heat the sausages until no longer pink; set aside.

Sauté the garlic and shallots in the same pan until they are softened; set aside.

Include the oyster sauce, pureed tomatoes, clam juice and wine; simmer for another 12 minutes.

Add the scallops, skinned sole and sausages. Let it simmer, partially covered, for another 6 minutes.

Enjoy garnished with fresh cilantro. Bon appétit!

NUTRITION: Calories 481, Protein 46.6g, Fat 26.9g, Carbs 5g, Sugar 1.1g

Hearty Chicken Rice Combo

Preparation time: 10 minutes Cooking Time: 10 minutes Servings: 6

INGREDIENTS:

- 12 ounces boneless, skinless chicken breast, cut into 12 strips
- Cooked white rice
- Juice of 2 limes
- 2 tbsps brown sugar
- 1 tbsp minced garlic
- 2 tsps ground cumin

DIRECTIONS:

In a mixing bowl, add lime juice, brown sugar, garlic, and cumin. Combine to mix well with each other.

Add chicken and combine well. Marinate for 1 hour in the refrigerator.

Remove chicken and thread into pre-soaked skewers.

Preheat grill over medium heat setting; grease grates with some oil.

Grill chicken 4 minutes each side until golden brown and juicy.

Serve warm with cooked rice.

Nutrition:

Calories: 93 Fat: 2g Phosphorus: 131mg Potassium: 233mg Sodium: 110mg Carbohydrates: 5g Protein: 12g

BAKED EGGPLANT TURKEY

Preparation time: 10 minutes Cooking Time: 50 minutes Servings: 6-8

INGREDIENTS:

- ½ cup green pepper, chopped
- ½ cup onion, finely chopped
- 1 large eggplant
- 2 tbsps vegetable oil
- 2 cups plain breadcrumbs
- 1 large egg, slightly beaten
- 1-pound lean ground turkey
- ½ tsp red pepper, optional

DIRECTIONS:

Preheat an oven to 350ºF. Grease a casserole dish with some cooking spray.

In boiling water, cook eggplant until fully tender.

Drain and mash eggplant well.

Take a medium saucepan or skillet, add oil. Heat over medium heat.

Add onion, green pepper, and stir-cook until it becomes translucent and softened.

Add ground meat and stir-cook until evenly brown.

Mix in eggplant, egg, and breadcrumbs. Season to taste with red pepper.

Add the mixture in a casserole dish and bake for 35-45 minutes until meat is cooked to satisfaction.

Serve warm.

Nutrition:

Calories 263, Fat 7g, Phosphorus 162mg, Potassium 373mg, Sodium 281mg, Carbohydrates 4g, Protein 14g

SCALLOP CEVICHE

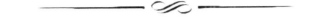

Preparation Time: 5 Minutes Cooking Time: 20 minutes Servings: 2

INGREDIENTS:

- 6 fresh scallops
- Juice of ½ lemon
- 1 tbsp olive oil with red pepper
- Few sprigs of fresh coriander
- 2 tbsp pomegranate seeds
- Optional: ½ finely chopped red pepper when you don't have spicy olive oil

DIRECTIONS:

Prepare a nice big plate. Then cut the scallops into three thin slices. Divide them over the plate and continue to flavor.

Drizzle the lemon juice and olive oil over the scallops. Add red pepper, Finish with coriander leaves, pomegranate seeds and a pinch of salt.

NUTRITION:

Calories 168.6, Total Fat 1.4 g, Saturated Fat 0.2 g, Polyunsaturated Fat 0.5 g, Monounsaturated Fat 0.1 g, Cholesterol 49.9 mg, Sodium 249.1 mg, Potassium 711.4 mg, Total Carbohydrate 13.0 g, Dietary Fiber 1.4 g, Sugars 1.2 g, Protein 26.4 g

ITALIAN TURKEY MEATLOAF

Preparation time: 10 minutes Cooking Time: 45 minutes Servings: 6-8

INGREDIENTS:

- ½ tsp Italian seasoning
- ¼ tsp black pepper
- ½ tsp onion powder
- ½ cup chopped onions
- 1-pound lean ground turkey
- 1 egg white
- 1 tbsp lemon juice
- ½ cup plain breadcrumbs
- ½ cup diced green bell pepper
- ¼ cup of water

DIRECTIONS:

Preheat an oven to 400ºF. Grease a baking dish with some cooking spray.

In a mixing bowl, add turkey and lemon juice. Combine to mix well with each other.

Add other ingredients and combine well.

Add the mixture in a baking dish and bake for 40-45 minutes until cooked to satisfaction.

Serve warm.

NUTRITION:

Calories 123, Fat 6g, Phosphorus 94mg, Potassium 142mg, Sodium 83mg, Carbohydrates 9g, Protein 13g

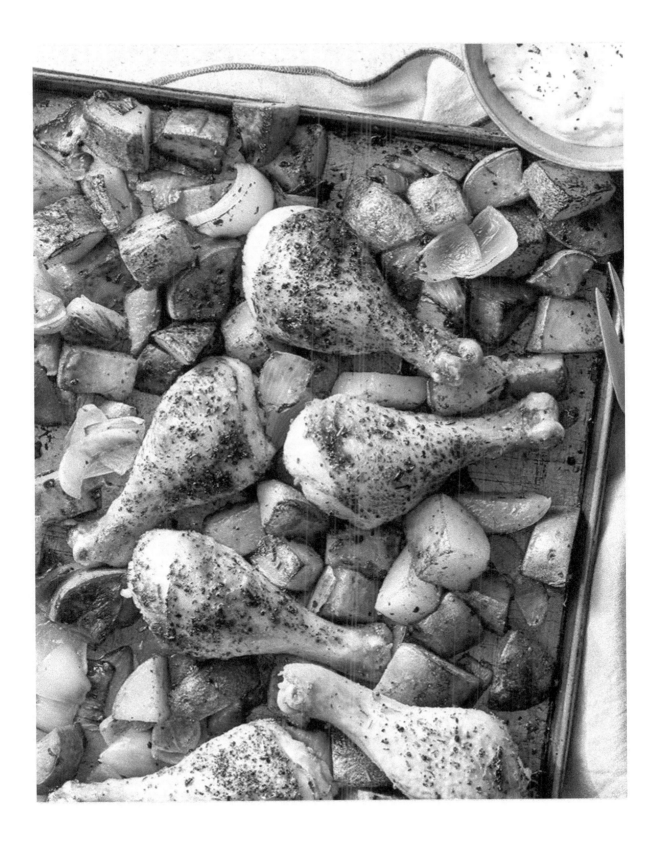

ROASTED CHICKEN DRUMSTICKS

Preparation Time: 15 minutes Cooking Time: 50 minutes Servings: 4-6

INGREDIENTS:

- 1 medium onion, chopped
- 1-2 tbsps fresh turmeric, chopped
- 1-2 tbsps fresh ginger, chopped
- 2 lemongrass stalks (bottom third), peeled and chopped
- 1-2 jalapeños, seeded and chopped
- 1 tsp fresh lime zest, grated
- 1 tbsp curry powder
- 1¼ cups unsweetened coconut milk
- 3 tbsps fresh lime juice
- 1 tbsp coconut aminos
- 1 tbsp fish sauce
- 4-pound chicken kegs
- Chopped fresh cilantro, for garnishing

DIRECTIONS:

In a blender, add all ingredients except chicken legs and pulse till smooth.

Transfer a combination in a large baking dish.

Add chicken and coat with marinade generously.

Cover and refrigerate to marinade approximately 12 hours.

Remove chicken from refrigerator and in room temperature approximately 25-half an hour before cooking.

Preheat the oven to 350F.

Uncover the baking dish and roast or about 50 minutes.

NUTRITION:

Calories 432, Fat 13g, Carbohydrates 19g, Fiber 6g, Protein 35g

GRILLED CHICKEN

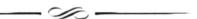

Preparation Time: 15 minutes Cooking Time: 41 minutes Servings: 4-6

INGREDIENTS:

- 1 (3-inch) piece fresh ginger, minced
- 6 small garlic cloves, minced
- 1½ tbsps tamarind paste
- 1 tbsp organic honey
- ¼ cup coconut aminos
- 2½ tbsps extra virgin olive oil
- 1½ tbsps sesame oil, toasted
- ½ tsp ground cardamom
- Salt and freshly ground white pepper, to taste
- 1 (4-5-pound) whole chicken, cut into 8 pieces

DIRECTIONS:

In a large glass bowl, mix together all ingredients except chicken pieces.

With a fork, pierce the chicken pieces completely.

Add chicken pieces in bowl and coat with marinade generously.

Cover and refrigerate to marinate for approximately a couple of hours to overnight.

Preheat the grill to medium heat. Grease the grill grate.

Place the chicken pieces on grill, bone-side down.

Grill covered approximately 20-25 minutes.

Change the side and grill, covered approximately 6-8 minutes.

Change alongside it and grill, covered for about 5-8 minutes.

NUTRITION:

Calories 423, Fat 12g, Carbohydrates 20g, Fiber 3g, Protein 42g

GRILLED CHICKEN BREAST

Preparation Time: 15 minutes Cooking Time: 20 minutes Servings: 4-6

INGREDIENTS:

- 2 scallions, chopped
- 1 (1-inch) piece fresh ginger, minced
- 2 minced garlic cloves
- 1 cup fresh pineapple juice
- ¼ cup coconut aminos
- ¼ cup extra-virgin organic olive oil
- 1 tsp ground cinnamon
- 1 tsp ground cumin
- 1 tsp ground turmeric
- Salt, to taste
- 4 skinless, boneless chicken breasts

DIRECTIONS:

Add all the ingredients to a big Ziploc bag and seal it.

Shake the bag to coat the chicken with marinade well.

Refrigerate to marinate for about twenty or so minutes to an hour.

Preheat the grill to medium-high heat. Grease the grill grate.

Place the chicken pieces on the grill and grill for about 10 min per side.

NUTRITION:

Calories 445, Fat 9g, Carbohydrates 21g, Fiber 4g, Protein 39g

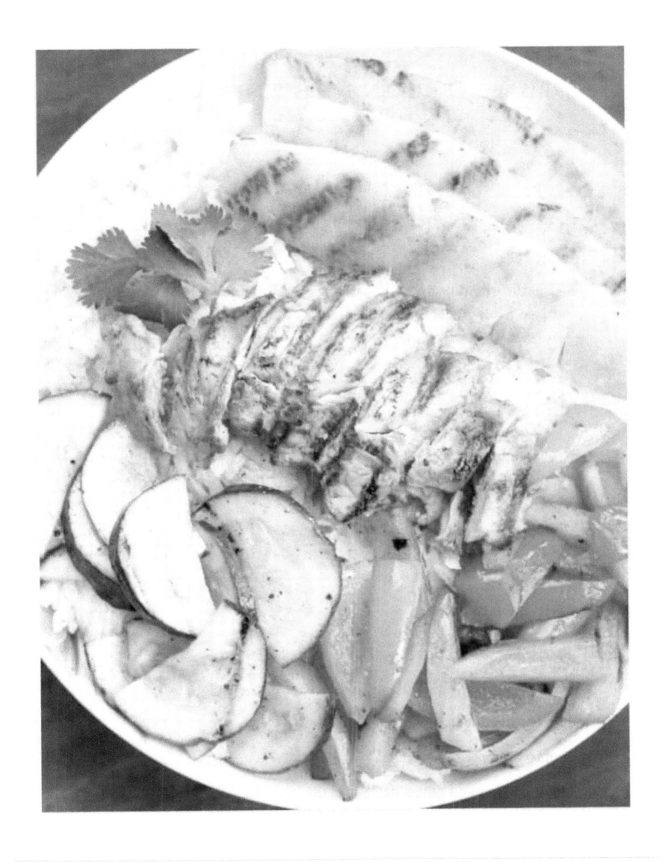

GRILLED CHICKEN WITH PINEAPPLE & VEGGIES

Preparation Time: 5 Minutes Cooking Time: 22 minutes Servings: 4-6

INGREDIENTS:

- For the sauce:
- 1 garlic oil, minced
- ¾ tsp fresh ginger, minced
- ½ cup coconut aminos
- ¼ cup fresh pineapple juice
- 2 tbsps freshly squeezed lemon juice
- 2 tbsps balsamic vinegar
- ¼ tsp red pepper flakes, crushed
- Salt and freshly ground black pepper, to taste
- For grilling:
- 4 skinless, boneless chicken breasts
- 1 pineapple, peeled and sliced
- 1 bell pepper, seeded and cubed
- 1 zucchini, sliced
- 1red onion, sliced

DIRECTIONS:

For the sauce - mix all ingredients in a pan on medium-high heat.

Bring to a boil reducing the heat to medium-low.

Cook approximately 5-6 minutes.

Remove from heat and put aside to cool down slightly.

Coat the chicken breasts with about ¼ of the sauce.

Keep aside for approximately half an hour.

Preheat the grill to medium-high heat. Grease the grill grate.

Place the chicken pieces on the grill and grill for around 5-8 minutes per side.

Now, squeeze the pineapple and vegetables on the grill grate.

Grill the pineapple for around 3 minutes per side.

Grill the vegetables for approximately 4-5 minutes, flipping them midway.

Cut the chicken breasts into desired size slices.

Distribute chicken, pineapple and vegetables onto serving plates.

Serve alongside the remaining sauce.

NUTRITION:

Calories 435, Fat 12g, Carbohydrates 25g, Fiber 13g, Protein 38g

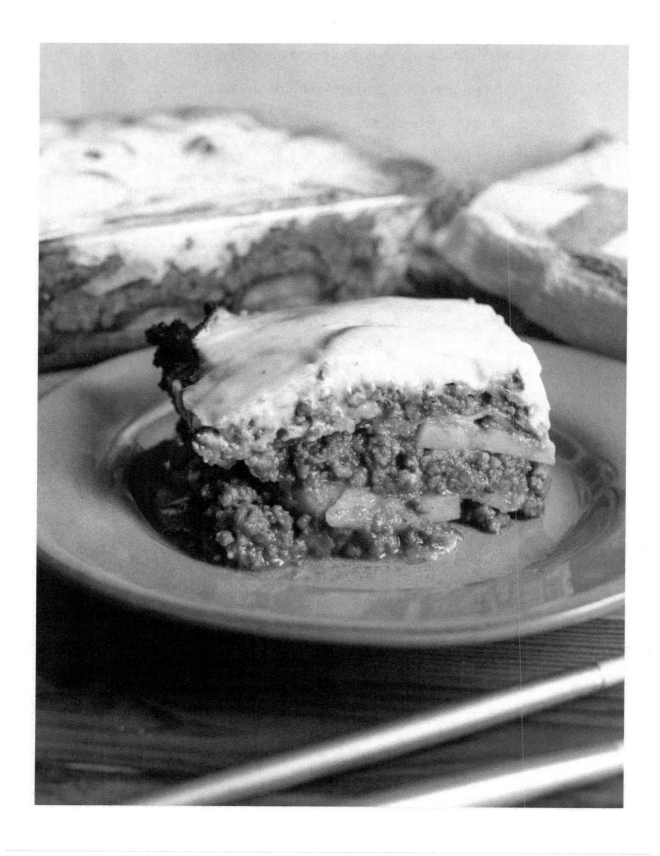

Light Paprika Moussaka

Preparation Time: 15 minutes Cooking time: 45 minutes Servings: 3

INGREDIENTS:

- 1 eggplant, trimmed
- 1 cup ground chicken
- 1/3 cup white onion, diced
- 3 oz Cheddar cheese, shredded
- 1 potato, sliced
- 1 tsp olive oil
- 1 tsp salt
- ½ cup milk
- 1 tbsp butter
- 1 tbsp ground paprika
- 1 tbsp Italian seasoning
- 1 tsp tomato paste

DIRECTIONS:

Slice the eggplant lengthwise and sprinkle with salt.

Pour olive oil in the skillet and add sliced potato.

Roast potato for 2 minutes from each side.

Then transfer it in the plate.

Put eggplant in the skillet and roast it for 2 minutes from each side too.

Pour milk in the pan and bring it to boil.

Add tomato paste, Italian seasoning, paprika, butter and Cheddar cheese.

Then mix up together onion with ground chicken.

Arrange the sliced potato in the casserole in one layer.

Then add ½ of all sliced eggplants.

Spread the eggplants with ½ of chicken mixture.

Then add the remaining eggplants.

Pour the milk mixture over the eggplants.

Bake moussaka for 30 minutes at 355F.

NUTRITION:

calories 387, fat 21.2g, fiber 8.9g, carbs 26.3g, protein 25.4g

YEAST DINNER ROLLS

Preparation Time: 5 Minutes Cooking Time: 20 minutes Servings: 4

INGREDIENTS:

- 1 cup hot water
- 6 tbsps vegetable shortening
- ½ cup sugar
- 1 package yeast
- 2 tbsps of warm water
- 1 egg
- 3 ¾ - 4 cup all-purpose flour

DIRECTIONS:

Preheat oven to 400°F.

Combine hot water, shortening and sugar in a large bowl. Set aside to cool to room temperature.

Dissolve yeast in warm water.

Add egg, yeast, and half the flour to the mixture in the large bowl. Beat well.

Stir in the remaining flour with a spoon until easy to handle.

Allow to rest 1 to 1 ½ hours or until the dough has doubled in size.

Cut off amount needed to shape rolls.

Bake rolls for 12 minutes or until done.

NUTRITION:

148 calories, 0grams trans-fat, 5mg Sodium, 3g protein, 12mg cholesterol, 31mg Potassium, 4g total fat, 24g carbohydrates, 32mg phosphorus, 1g saturated fat, 1g fiber, 5mg Calcium

CUCUMBER BOWL WITH SPICES AND GREEK YOGURT

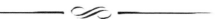

Preparation Time: 10 minutes Cooking time: 20 minutes Servings: 3

INGREDIENTS:

- 4 cucumbers
- ½ tsp chili pepper
- ¼ cup fresh parsley, chopped
- ¾ cup fresh dill, chopped
- 2 tbsps lemon juice
- ½ tsp salt
- ½ tsp ground black pepper
- ¼ tsp sage
- ½ tsp dried oregano
- 1/3 cup Greek yogurt

DIRECTIONS:

Make the cucumber dressing: blend the dill and parsley until you get green mash.

Then combine together green mash with lemon juice, salt, ground black pepper, sage, dried oregano, Greek yogurt and chili pepper.

Churn the mixture well.

Chop the cucumbers roughly and combine them with cucumber dressing. Mix well.

Refrigerate the cucumber for 20 minutes.

NUTRITION:

calories 114, fat 1.6g, fiber 4.1g, carbs 23.2g, protein 7.6g

STUFFED BELL PEPPERS WITH QUINOA

Preparation Time: 10 minutes Cooking time: 35 minutes Servings: 2

INGREDIENTS:

- 2 bell peppers
- 1/3 cup quinoa
- 3 oz chicken stock
- ¼ cup onion, diced
- ½ tsp salt
- ¼ tsp tomato paste
- ½ tsp dried oregano
- 1/3 cup sour cream
- 1 tsp paprika

DIRECTIONS:

Trim the bell peppers and remove the seeds.

Then combine together chicken stock and quinoa in the pan.

Add salt and boil the ingredients for 10 minutes or until quinoa will soak all liquid.

Then combine together cooked quinoa with dried oregano, tomato paste, and onion.

Fill the bell peppers with the quinoa mixture and arrange in the casserole mold.

Add sour cream and bake the peppers for 25 minutes at 365F.

Serve the cooked peppers with sour cream sauce from the casserole mold.

NUTRITION:

Calories 237, fat 10.3g, fiber 4.5g, carbs 31.3g, protein 6.9g

Mediterranean Burrito

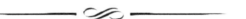

Preparation Time: 10 minutes Cooking Time: 20 minutes Servings: 4

INGREDIENTS:

- 2 wheat tortillas
- 2 oz red kidney beans, canned, drained
- 2 tbsps hummus
- 2 tsps tahini sauce
- 1 cucumber
- 2 lettuce leaves
- 1 tbsp lime juice
- 1 tsp olive oil
- ½ tsp dried oregano

DIRECTIONS:

Mash the red kidney beans until you get a puree.

Then spread the wheat tortillas with beans mash from one side.

Add hummus and tahini sauce.

Cut the cucumber into the wedges and place them over tahini sauce.

Then add lettuce leaves.

Make the dressing: mix up together olive oil, dried oregano, and lime juice.

Drizzle the lettuce leaves with the dressing and wrap the wheat tortillas in the shape of burritos.

NUTRITION: calories 288, fat 10.2g, fiber 14.6g, carbs 38.2g, protein 12.5g

Chapter 8: Snacks and desserts

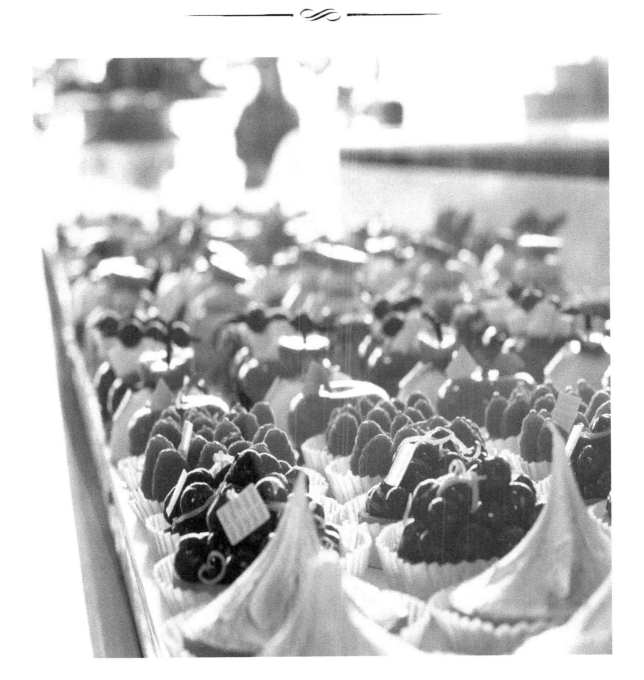

Snacks and desserts

194. PECAN PANCAKE

195. LEMON SQUARES

196. HOMEMADE APPLESAUCE

197. ICE CREAM SANDWICHES

199. BLACKBERRY MOUNTAIN PIE

200. CREAMY PINEAPPLE DESSERT

201. CHOCOLATE GELATIN MOUSSE

202. BLACKBERRY CREAM CHEESE PIE

203. BLUEBERRY MUFFINS

204. UPLAND CRESS AND CAULIFLOWER OPEN-FACED SANDWICH

205. OVEN BAKED EGGPLANT FRIES

206. GLUTEN-FREE DARK CHOCO ALMOND BUTTER

207. MANGO PEAR SALSA

208. ZUCCHINI CHIPS

209. CARROT MUFFIN CAKE

210. BERRY FRUIT SALAD WITH YOGURT

211. BLUEBERRY BAKED BREAD

212. HERB BREAD

SNACKS AND DESSERTS

PECAN PANCAKE

Servings: 4 Time: 15 Minutes

INGREDIENTS:

- 4 cups pecan flour, finely milled, add more later for kneading
- 2 ½ cups water
- ½ cup cilantro leaves, minced
- ½ cup coconut oil
- Pinch of kosher salt
- For the Dipping Sauce
- Low-sodium salsa, store-bought

DIRECTIONS:

1. Combine dipping sauce in a small bowl. Set aside.

2. Lightly grease a large nonstick skillet with coconut oil; set aside.

3. Mix remaining ingredients in a bowl until dough comes together. Turn out dough on lightly floured flat surface; knead until elastic. Divide into 8 equal portions; roll into balls, tucking in edges underneath to make dough look seamless. Using a rolling pin, flatten each out to roughly the size of skillet's cooking surface.

4. Set skillet over medium heat. Fry flatbreads one at a time until small pockets of air develop within; flip and continue cooking until lightly brown on both sides. Place cooked pieces on a serving platter lined with tea towel.

5. Using pastry brush, lightly grease both sides of the flatbread with oil. Cover platter with another tea towel to prevent bread from drying out. Repeat step until all flat breads are cooked.

6. Place 2 pieces on plates; slice these into wedges. Serve with desired amount of

dipping sauce on the side.

Nutrition:

Protein 4.62g (8%), Potassium (K) 218 mg (5%), Sodium (Na) 48mg (28%)

LEMON SQUARES

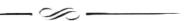

Preparation time: 10 minutes Cooking Time: 35 minutes Servings: 12

INGREDIENTS:

- 1 cup powdered sugar
- 1 cup all-purpose white flour
- ½ cup unsalted butter
- 1 cup granulated sugar
- ½ tsp baking powder
- 2 eggs, slightly beaten
- 4 tbsps lemon juice
- 1 tbsp unsalted butter, softened
- 1 tbsp lemon rind, grated

DIRECTIONS:

Start mixing ¼ cup confectioner's sugar, ½ cup butter, and flour in a bowl.

Spread this crust mixture in an 8-inch square pan and press it.

Bake this flour crust for 15 minutes at 350°F.

Meanwhile, prepare the filling by beating granulated sugar, 2 tablespoons lemon juice, lemon rind, eggs and baking powder in a mixer.

Spread this filling in the baked crust and bake again for 20 minutes.

Prepare the icing meanwhile by beating 1 tablespoon butter with 2 tablespoons lemon juice and ¾ cup confectioners' sugar.

Once the lemon pie is baked, allow it to cool.

Drizzle the icing mixture on top of the lemon pie then cut it into 36 squares.

Serve.

NUTRITION:

Calories 146, Protein 2g, Carbohydrates 22g, Fat 6g, Cholesterol 39mg, Sodium 45mg, Potassium 22mg, Phosphorus 32mg, Calcium 16mg, Fiber 0.2g

HOMEMADE APPLE SAUCE

Preparation time: 5 minutes Cooking time: 40 minutes Servings: 3

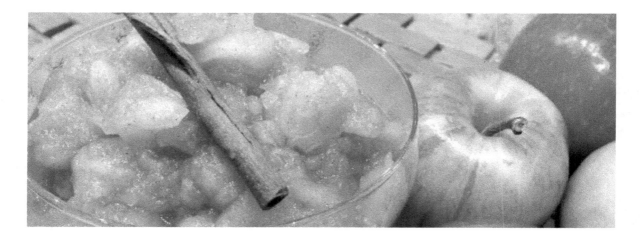

INGREDIENTS:

- 6 pounds of apples, peeled, cored and cut into 8 slices
- 1 cup apple juice or apple cider
- 1 lemon (juice)
- ½ tsp brown sugar
- 1 tsp of cinnamon (more or less to taste)

DIRECTIONS:

Combine all the ingredients in a large saucepan and cook over medium heat, stirring occasionally for 25 minutes.

Mash gently in a food processor or blender (do not overfill; divide into two portions if necessary) until smooth.

NUTRITION:

Calories 124kcal, Potassium 182mg, Sodium 3mg, Phosphorus 20mg, Protein 1g

ICE CREAM SANDWICHES

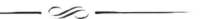

Preparation time: 5 minutes Cooking time: 30 minutes Servings: 3

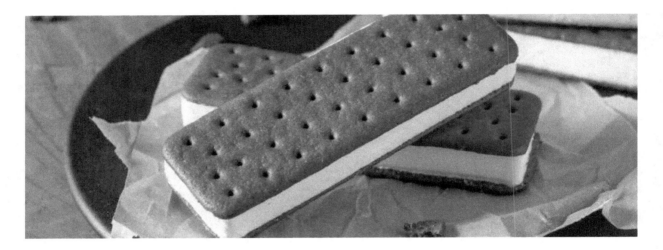

INGREDIENTS:

- 10 easy graham crackers
- 20 tbsps nondairy whisk, fresh

DIRECTIONS

Break the graham crackers in half.

Put 2 tablespoons cold whisk into each half.

Cover with the other half of the cookie.

Place on the dish and freeze for several hours.

Wrap individual frozen rolls in Saran Wrap.

Nutrition:

Calories 37kcal, Potassium 18mg, Sodium 36mg, Phosphorus 15mg, Protein 1g

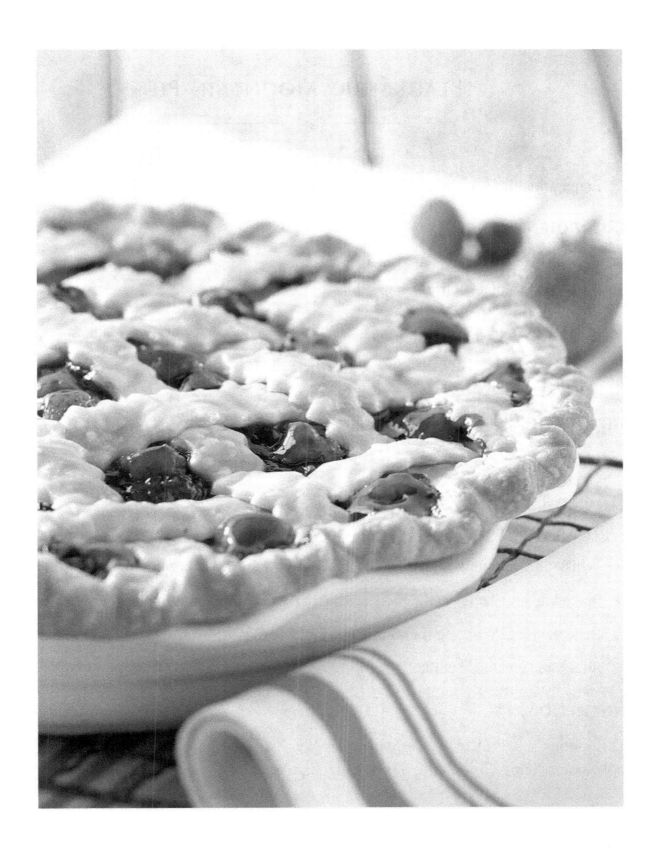

BLACKBERRY MOUNTAIN PIE

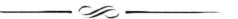

Preparation time: 10 minutes Cooking Time: 45 minutes Servings: 8

INGREDIENTS:

- 1/3 cup unsalted butter
- 4 cups blackberries
- 13 tbsps sugar
- 1 cup all-purpose white flour
- ½ tsp baking powder
- ¾ cup Rice Drink

DIRECTION:

Preheat oven to 375°F.

Grease a 2-quart baking dish with melted butter.

Toss blackberries with 1 tablespoon sugar in a small bowl.

Whisk the remaining ingredients in a mixer until they form a smooth batter.

Spread this pie batter in the prepared baking dish and top it with blackberries.

Bake the blackberry pie for 45 minutes in the preheated oven.

Slice and serve once chilled.

NUTRITION:

Calories 320, Protein 4g, Carbohydrates 49g, Fat 12g, Cholesterol 28mg, Sodium 222mg, Potassium 186mg, Phosphorus 91mg, Calcium 65mg, Fiber 5.6g

CREAMY PINEAPPLE DESSERT

Preparation time: 10 minutes Cooking Time: 0 minutes Servings: 2

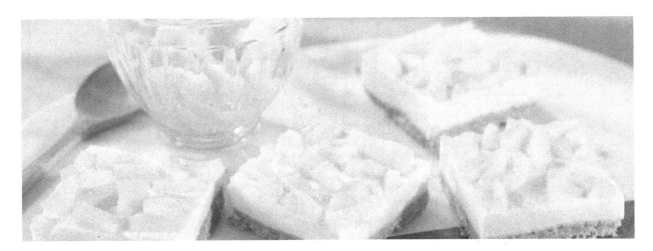

Ingredients:

- 16 ounces cottage cheese
- 15 ounces canned pineapple
- 8 ounces whipped topping
- ½ tsp green food coloring

DIRECTION:

Throw all the dessert ingredients into a suitably sized bowl.

Mix them well and refrigerate for 1 hour.

Serve.

NUTRITION:

Calories 204, Protein 10g, Carbohydrates 23g, Fat 8g, Cholesterol 13mg, Sodium 303mg, Potassium 203mg, Phosphorus 152mg, Calcium 100mg, Fiber 0.6g

CHOCOLATE GELATIN MOUSSE

Preparation time: 10 minutes Cooking time: 5 minutes Servings: 4

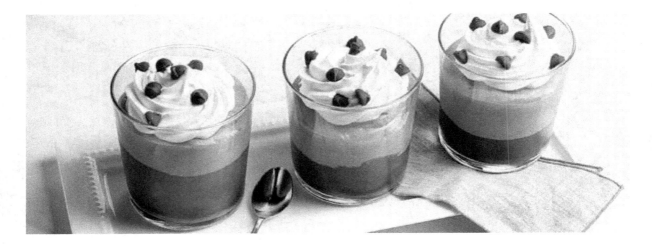

INGREDIENTS:

- 1 tsp stevia
- ½ tsp gelatin
- ¼ cup milk
- ½ cup chocolate chips
- 1 tsp vanilla
- ½ cup heavy cream, whipped

DIRECTIONS:

Whisk the stevia with the gelatin and milk in a saucepan and cook up to a boil.

Stir in the chocolate and vanilla, then mix well until it has completely melted.

Beat the cream in a mixer until fluffy then fold in the chocolate mixture.

Mix it gently with a spatula then transfer to the serving bowl.

Refrigerate the dessert for 4 hours.

Serve.

NUTRITION:

Calories 200, Total Fat 12.1g, Saturated Fat 8g, Cholesterol 27mg, Sodium 31mg, Carbohydrates 4.7g, Dietary Fiber 0.7g, Sugars 0.8g, Protein 3.2g, Calcium 68mg, Phosphorus 120mg, Potassium 100mg

BLACKBERRY CREAM CHEESE PIE

Preparation time: 10 minutes Cooking time: 45 minutes Servings: 8

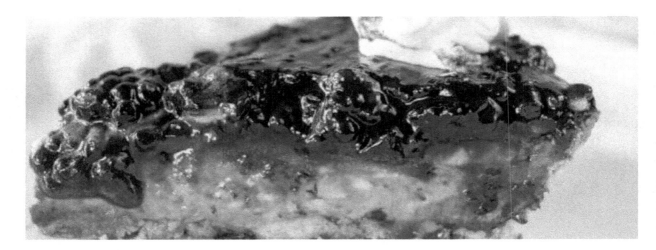

INGREDIENTS:

- 1/3 cup butter, unsalted
- 4 cups blackberries
- 1 tsp stevia
- 1 cup flour
- ½ tsp baking powder
- ¾ cup cream cheese

DIRECTIONS:

Preheat the oven to 375F.

Layer a 2-quart baking dish with melted butter.

Mix the blackberries with stevia in a small bowl.

Beat the remaining ingredients in a mixer until they form a smooth batter.

Evenly spread this pie batter in the prepared baking dish and top it with blackberries.

Bake the blackberry pie for about 45 minutes in the preheated oven.

Slice and serve once chilled.

NUTRITION:

Calories 239, Total Fat 8.4g, Saturated Fat 4.9g, Cholesterol 20mg, Sodium 63mg, Carbohydrates 26.2g, Dietary Fiber 4.5g, Sugars 15.1g, Protein 2.8g, Calcium 67mg, Phosphorus 105mg, Potassium 170mg

BLUEBERRY MUFFINS

Preparation time: 10 minutes Cooking time: 15 minutes Servings: 6

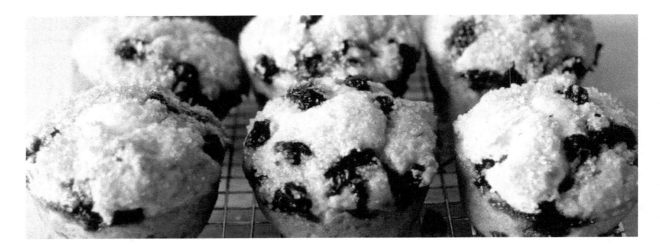

INGREDIENTS

- 1 egg white
- ¼ cup margarine
- ½ cup sugar
- 7 tbsps water
- ½ tsp vanilla extract
- 1 tsp baking powder
- 1 cup all-purpose flour
- 1 cup blueberries, canned and drained or fresh

DIRECTIONS

Preheat oven to 375ºF.

Beat egg white in a small mixing bowl until stiff. Set aside.

Cream margarine and sugar together until smooth.

Add water and vanilla, mixing thoroughly.

Add baking powder and flour.

Fold in beaten egg white and blueberries.

Bake in greased muffin pan for 30 minutes.

Nutrition:

0g trans-fat, 139mg sodium, 1.5g protein, 0mg cholesterol, 71mg potassium, 4g total fat, 21g carbohydrate, 94mg phosphorus, 0g saturated fat, 1g fiber, 29mg calcium

Upland Cress and Cauliflower Open-Faced Sandwich

Preparation time: 5 Minutes Cooking Time: 30 Minutes Servings: 3

INGREDIENTS:

- 1 slice, thick sugar-free pumpernickel bread, toasted
- 1 handful, generous upland cress, thin stems and leaves only, add more if desired (substitute alfalfa sprouts, arugula leaves, or watercress)
- ½ cup cooked, chopped cauliflower
- 1 tsp heaped Colby Jack cheese, grated
- ¼ tsp balsamic vinegar, for drizzling

DIRECTIONS:

Spread mashed avocado on 1 side of bread. Place upland cress on top.

Drizzle balsamic vinegar before sprinkling cheese on top.

Heat open-faced sandwich in oven toaster until cheese melts.

Cool slightly before slicing. Slice diagonally in half. Serve.

NUTRITION:

Protein 4.63g, Potassium (K) 145 mg, Sodium (Na) 172 mg

Oven Baked Eggplant Fries

Preparation time: 5 Minutes Cooking Time: 40 Minutes Servings: 3

INGREDIENTS:

- 1 large eggplant
- 1 low sodium veggie broth
- ½ tsp of ground black pepper
- 1 tsp of smoked paprika
- 2 tsps of stevia
- 1 cup of almond meal
- 2 tbsps of nutritional yeast
- 1 tbsp of lemon juice

DIRECTIONS:

Preheat your oven to a temperature of 400°F

Wash the eggplants and cut them into thin sticks.

Put the eggplant pieces in a medium bowl; then sprinkle with veggie broth, lemon juice, pepper, paprika and stevia. Mix well.

Place the almond meal and nutritional yeast in a separate bowl and mix your ingredients well; then place the eggplant pieces in a bowl with almond meal; toss well.

Place the eggplant pieces over a baking sheet covered with parchment paper.

Bake the eggplant pieces in a preheated oven for about 40 minutes

Serve and enjoy your oven baked eggplant pieces!

NUTRITION: Calories 166, Fats 11.7g, Carbs 6g, Fiber 1.3g, Potassium 104mg, Sodium 99mg, Phosphorus 75mg, Protein 9g

Gluten-free Dark Choco Almond Butter

Preparation time: 5 Minutes Cooking Time: 20 Minutes Servings: 3

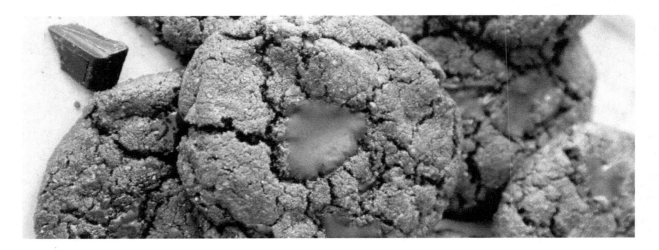

INGREDIENTS:

- ½ tsp baking soda
- 1 cup almond butter
- 1 egg, large
- ¾ cup sugar
- ½ tsp salt
- ½ cup dark chocolate, chopped

DIRECTIONS:

Preheat the oven to 350°F. Line a baking sheet.

Meanwhile, put together baking soda, almond butter, egg, sugar and salt. Mix until all ingredients are well-combined.

Fold in the chocolate. Mix until it forms a dough.

Spoon an equal amount of mixture on a baking sheet. Place inside the oven and bake for 10 minutes.

Allow cookies to cool before serving.

NUTRITION:

Protein 7.83g, Potassium (K) 288 mg, Sodium (Na) 237mg

MANGO PEAR SALSA

Preparation time: 5 Minutes Cooking Time: 40 Minutes Servings: 3

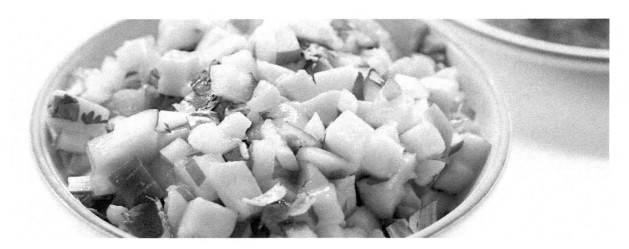

INGREDIENTS:

- 1 mango, chunked
- ¼ cup red onion, finely chopped
- 2 pears, cored, chunked
- ¼ cup yellow bell pepper, finely chopped
- ¼ cup red bell pepper, finely chopped
- 2 tsp olive oil
- 3 tbsps fresh cilantro, chopped
- 1 jalapeño pepper, finely chopped
- Pinch of salt
- 1 tbsp lime juice

DIRECTIONS:

Mix mango, red onion, pears, yellow bell pepper, red bell pepper, olive oil, cilantro, jalapeño pepper, salt and lime juice in a bowl. Mix well until all ingredients are well combined. Wrap the bowl.

Place inside the refrigerator. Serve as needed.

NUTRITION:

Protein 0.77g, Potassium (K) 171 mg and Sodium (Na) 22mg

ZUCCHINI CHIPS

Preparation time: 5 Minutes Cooking Time: 20 Minutes Servings: 3

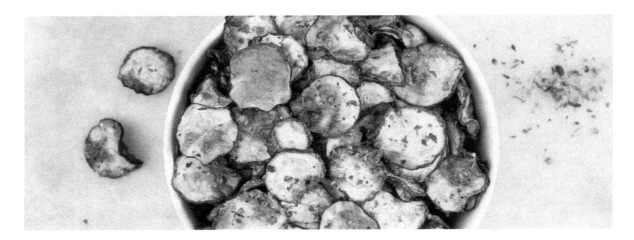

INGREDIENTS:

- 4 zucchinis, sliced thinly, ends removed
- 2 tbsps apple cider vinegar
- 2 tbsps olive oil
- ¼ tsp salt
- ¼ tsp ground black pepper

DIRECTIONS:

Preheat the oven to 225°F. Line a baking dish with parchment paper.

In a small bowl, pour vinegar, oil, salt, and pepper. Add zucchini. Mix all ingredients until the zucchini slices are well coated.

Layer coated zucchini in baking sheets. Place inside the oven. Bake for 2 hours.

Remove zucchini chips and let cool. Serve as needed. Leftovers can be stored in an airtight container.

Nutrition:

Protein 2.39g, Potassium (K) 519 mg and Sodium (Na) 162 mg, without added salt content of sodium is 16 mg

CARROT MUFFIN CAKE

Preparation time: 5 Minutes Cooking Time: 40 Minutes Servings: 3

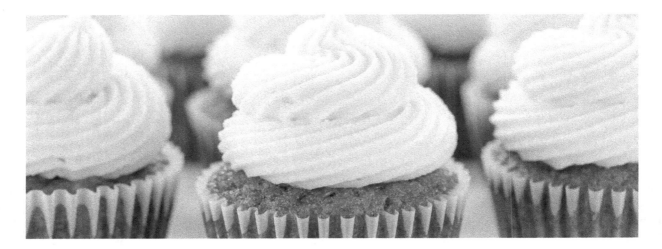

INGREDIENTS:

- 3 carrots, grated
- 5 pitted dates
- 1 cup lemon butter
- 1 egg
- 1 banana, mashed
- 2 tbsps melted butter
- 1 tsp nutmeg
- 1/3 cup almond flour
- Pinch of salt
- 1 tsp blackstrap molasses
- 1 tsp apple cider vinegar
- ½ tsp baking soda

DIRECTIONS:

Preheat the oven to 350°F. Line a muffin pan with parchment paper.

Combine egg, butter, banana, dates, nutmeg and molasses in a bowl. Stir well until all ingredients are well combined.

Tip in almond flour, baking soda and apple cider vinegar. Mix. Scatter carrots into the mixture.

Spoon batter into the prepared muffin pan. Place inside the oven. Bake for 25 minutes. Allow to cool before serving.

Nutrition:

Protein 1.54g, Potassium (K) 149 mg and Sodium (Na) 84 mg

BERRY FRUIT SALAD WITH YOGURT

Preparation time: 10 minutes Cooking time: 10 minutes Servings: 8

INGREDIENTS:

- ¼ cup honey
- 2 cups Greek yogurt
- 1 tbsp lemon juice
- 1 cup blackberries
- 1 cup red cherries, pitted and halved
- 1 cup blueberries
- 1 cup raspberries
- 2 tbsp honey

DIRECTIONS:

Combine the berries with the honey in a bowl.

Mix the yogurt, lemon juice, and honey in a separate bowl.

Place yogurt cream into the center of each glass.

Garnish with the berry fruit salad.

NUTRITION:

Protein 3.7g, Carbohydrates 27g, Fat 0.4g, Calories 117

BLUEBERRY BAKED BREAD

Preparation time: 5 Minutes Cooking Time: 30 Minutes Servings: 3

INGREDIENTS

- 1-quart blueberries, fresh or frozen
- ¼ cup water (omit if berries are frozen)
- 1 tsp lemon juice
- ½ cup sugar
- 1 pinch nutmeg
- 1 pinch cinnamon
- 1 tbsp margarine
- 3 slices bread, buttered and sprinkled with cinnamon and sugar on both sides

DIRECTIONS

Heat oven to 425°F.

Wash blueberries under cool running water.

Combine all ingredients except bread in a saucepan. Bring to a boil.

Pour blueberry mixture into a shallow baking pan; top with bread cut in halves.

Bake until brown (about 10 minutes).

NUTRITION:

176 calories, 0grams trans-fat, 92mg sodium, 2g protein, 0mg cholesterol, 83mg potassium, 3g total fat, 39g carbohydrates, 20mg phosphorus, 0g saturated fat, 3g fiber, 56mg calcium

HERB BREAD

Preparation time: 5 Minutes Cooking Time: 40 Minutes Servings: 3

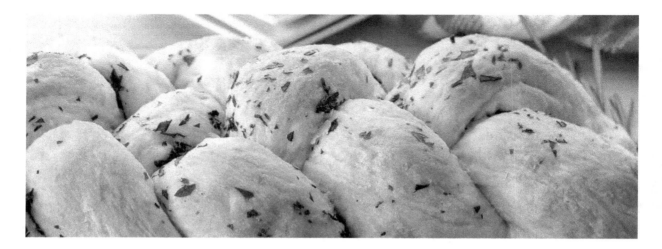

INGREDIENTS

- 1 loaf French bread
- ¼ cup margarine (unsalted)
- 2 tbsps chopped green onions
- 1 tsp thyme
- ¼ tsp tarragon
- 1 tsp basil flakes (optional)
- ½ tsp crushed marjoram (optional)

DIRECTIONS

Heat oven to 350°F.

Slice French bread almost to the bottom crust.

Combine margarine with remaining Ingredients.

Spread butter mixture on cut surfaces or slices using a brush.

Place on a baking sheet or pan.

Bake for 15-20 minutes.

NUTRITION:

120 calories, 0g trans-fat, 208mg sodium, 4g protein, 44mg potassium, 0mg cholesterol, 4g total fat, 18g carbohydrates, 37mg phosphorus, 1g saturated fat, 1g fiber, 15mg calcium

OATMEAL BERRY MUFFINS

Preparation time: 5 minutes Cooking time: 30 minutes Servings: 12

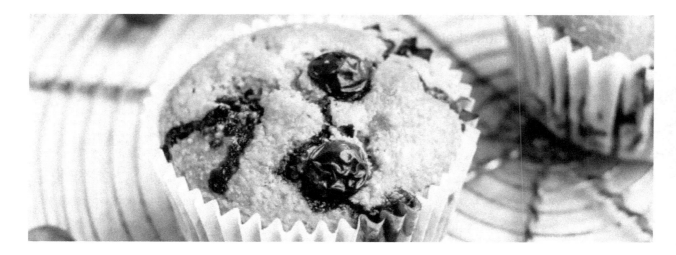

INGREDIENTS:

- ½ cup quick-cooking oatmeal
- 1 cup unbleached all-purpose flour
- ½ tsp baking soda
- ⅔ cup lightly packed brown sugar
- ½ cup applesauce
- 2 eggs
- Zest of 1 orange
- ¼ cup canola oil
- 1 tbsp lemon juice
- Zest of 1 lemon
- ¾ cup blueberries, fresh or frozen
- ¾ cup raspberries, fresh or frozen

Directions:

Preheat the oven to 350°F. Line 12 muffin cups.

Combine baking soda, brown sugar, oatmeal, and flour in a bowl. Set aside.

Whisk lemon juice, applesauce, and eggs in a large bowl.

Stir in the dry ingredients with wooden spoon.

Add the berries. Stir gently.

Scoop into the muffin cups.

Bake for 21 minutes. Let cool.

NUTRITION:

Protein 2.8g, Carbohydrates 28g, Fat 5.9g, Calories 173

AMBROSIA

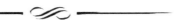

Preparation time: 1 hour Cooking time: 25 minutes Servings: 12

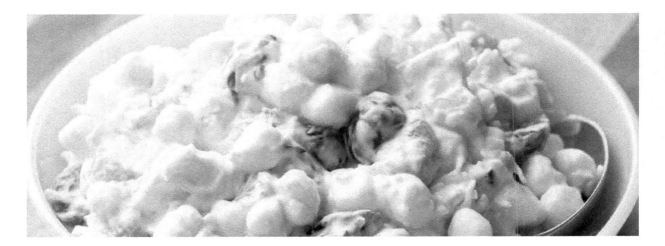

INGREDIENTS:

- ½ cup powdered sugar
- 1 cup sour cream
- 15 ounces canned pineapple chunks
- ½ tsp vanilla extract
- 1-½ cup maraschino cherries
- 15 ounces canned sliced peaches
- 3 cups miniature marshmallows

DIRECTIONS:

Mix vanilla, powdered sugar, and sour cream in a bowl.

Drain cherries, peaches, and pineapple.

Add marshmallows and fruits to sour cream mixture.

Let chill for an hour.

Serve.

NUTRITION:

Protein 1g, Carbohydrates 36g, Fat 4g, Calories 176

APPLE BARS

Preparation time: 15 minutes Cooking time: 50 minutes Servings: 18

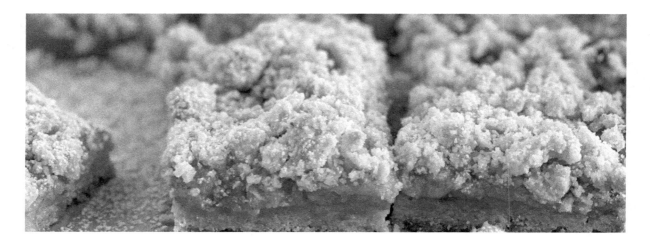

INGREDIENTS:

- ¾ cup unsalted butter
- 2 medium apples
- 1 cup sour cream
- 1 cup granulated sugar
- 1 tsp baking soda
- 1 tsp vanilla extract
- 2 cups all-purpose flour
- ½ tsp salt
- 1 tsp cinnamon
- ½ cup brown sugar
- 1 cup powdered sugar
- 2 tbsp milk

DIRECTIONS:

Preheat the oven to 350°F.

Chop and peel the apples.

Cream together ½ cup the granulated sugar and the butter.

Add flour, salt, baking soda, vanilla and sour cream. Stir to mix.

Add apples.

Pour the batter into a greased 9x13-inch baking pan.

Put cinnamon, brown sugar and 2 tablespoons of softened butter in a small bowl.

Bake for 40 minutes.

Let it cool and cut in 18 bars.

Nutrition:

Protein 2g, Carbohydrates 35g, Fat 11g, Calories 246

Chocolaty Chia Pudding

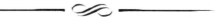

Preparation Time: 15 minutes Cooking Time: 20 minutes Servings: 4

INGREDIENTS:

6-9 dates, pitted and chopped

1½ cups unsweetened almond milk

1/3 cup chia seeds

¼ cup unsweetened cocoa powder

½ tsp ground cinnamon

Salt, to taste

½ tsp vanilla flavor

Directions:

In a mixer, add all ingredients and pulse till smooth.

Transfer the mixture into serving bowls.

Refrigerate to chill completely before serving.

NUTRITION:

Calories 166, Fat 7g, Carbohydrates 21g, Fiber 7g, Protein 17g

EGG CUSTARD

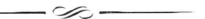

Preparation time: 8-10 minutes Cooking Time:20-30 minutes Servings: 4

INGREDIENTS:

- 3 tbsps sugar
- 1 tsp vanilla or lemon extract
- 1 tsp nutmeg
- 2 medium eggs
- ¼ cup almond or rice milk

DIRECTIONS:

Preheat an oven to 325°F.Grease 4 muffin pans or custard cups with some cooking spray.

In a mixing bowl, add all ingredients except nutmeg. Combine to mix well with each other.

Add the mixture in the pans, sprinkle nutmeg on top, and bake for 20-30 minutes until inserted toothpick comes out clean.

Serve warm.

NUTRITION:

Calories 82, Fat 3g, Phosphorus 46mg, Potassium 34mg, Sodium 41mg, Carbohydrates 13g, Protein 3g

Chocolate & Coffee Mousse

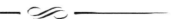

Preparation Time: 15 minutes Cooking Time: 20 minutes Servings: 4

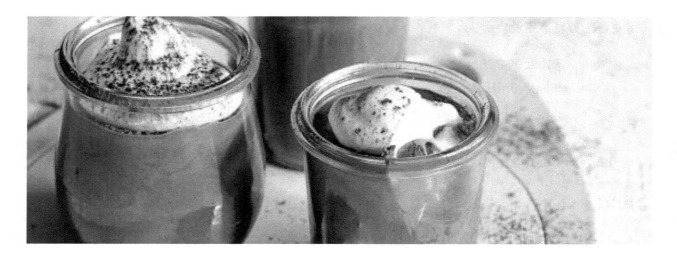

INGREDIENTS:

- ¼ cup chocolate brown chips
- ½ cup coconut milk
- ¼ cup boiling water
- 1 tbsp ground coffees
- Raw honey, to taste
- ¼ tsp almond extract
- 1 tbsp vanilla flavor

DIRECTIONS:

In a nonstick pan, add chocolate chips on medium-low heat.

Cook, stirring continuously for around 2-3 minutes or until the chocolate chips are melted.

Add coconut milk and beat till well combined.

Cook, stirring continuously for around 1-2 minutes.

Meanwhile, mix together hot water and coffee beans in a small bowl.

In a sizable bowl, add chocolate mixture, coffee mixture, honey and both extracts and mix till well combined.

Transfer the mousse into 4 serving glasses.

Refrigerate for approximately 2-3 hours.

NUTRITION:

Calories 112, Fat 3g, Carbohydrates 12g, Fiber 1g, Protein 2g

CHOCOLATY AVOCADO MOUSSE

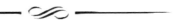

Preparation Time: 10 minutes Cooking Time: 20 minutes Servings: 4

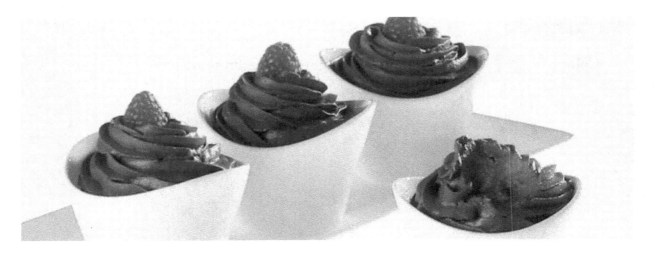

INGREDIENTS:

- 2 ripe avocados, peeled, pitted and chopped
- ½ cup coconut milk
- ½ cup cacao powder
- 1 tsp ground cinnamon
- ¼ tsp ground ancho Chile
- 1/3 cup raw honey
- 2 tsps vanilla extract

DIRECTIONS:

In a blender, add all ingredients and pulse till smooth.

Transfer the mousse in serving glasses.

Refrigerate to relax completely.

NUTRITION:

Calories 132, Fat 5g, Carbohydrates 26g, Fiber 6g, Protein 34g

Carrot Chia Pudding

Preparation Time: 15 minutes Cooking Time: 7 minutes Servings: 4

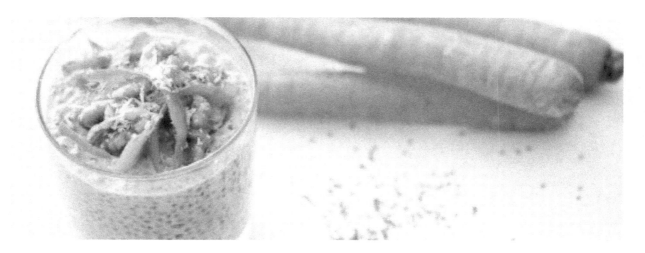

INGREDIENTS:

- ¾ cup carrot, peeled and chopped roughly
- 2-3 tbsps walnuts, chopped
- ½ tsp ground cinnamon
- ¼ tsp ground ginger
- Pinch of ground nutmeg
- Pinch of ground cloves
- 1-2 tbsps raw honey
- 1 cup unsweetened almond milk
- ½ cup water
- ½ tsp vanilla flavoring
- 2 tbsps chia seeds

DIRECTIONS:

In a mixer, add carrot and walnuts and pulse till chopped finely.

Transfer the carrot mixture in the nonstick pan on medium heat.

Add spices and honey and cook, stirring occasionally for about 5-7 minutes.

Stir in almond milk, water and vanilla extract.

Transfer a combination into a serving bowl.

Add chia seeds and stir to blend well.

NUTRITION:

Calories 137, Fat 2g, Carbohydrates 24g, Fiber 9g, Protein 6g

APPLE CHIA PUDDING

Preparation Time: 15 minutes Cooking Time: 20 minutes Servings: 4

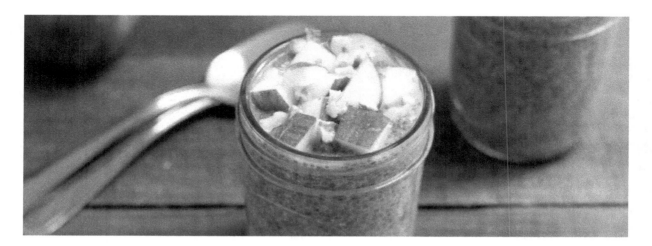

INGREDIENTS:

- ½ cup unsweetened almond milk
- 2 tbsps chia seeds
- ½ tsp ground cinnamon, divided
- 1/8 tsp vanilla extract
- 1 apple, cored and chopped finely
- ½ tsp raw honey
- 1½ tsps water
- 2 tbsps golden raisins

DIRECTIONS:

In a bowl, mix together almond milk, chia seeds, ¼ tsp of cinnamon and vanilla flavoring.

Refrigerate for around 1-120 minutes.

In a microwave safe bowl, mix together apple, honey, water and remaining cinnamon and microwave on high for around 1-2 minutes, stirring once.

Remove from microwave and stir in raisins.

Add 50 % of apple mixture in chia seeds mixture and stir to blend.

Refrigerate before serving.

Top with remaining apple mixture and serve.

NUTRITION:

Calories 123, Fat 3g, Carbohydrates 15g, Fiber 4g, Protein 6g

ROSEMARY FLATBREAD

Preparation time: 3 hours Cooking time: 20 minutes Servings: 12

INGREDIENTS:

- 3 cups coconut flour, finely milled
- 2 ½ cups water
- 1 cup all-purpose flour
- ½ cup fresh rosemary, minced
- ½ cup coconut oil, melted
- Pinch of kosher salt
- For the Dipping Sauce:
- ¼ pound ripe tomatoes, minced
- ¼ tsp pomegranate vinegar
- Pinch of Himalayan pink salt
- Pinch of white pepper

DIRECTIONS:

1. Combine dipping sauce in small bowl. Set aside.

2. Lightly grease a large nonstick skillet with coconut oil; set aside.

3. Mix remaining ingredients in a bowl until dough comes together. Turn out dough on lightly floured flat surface; knead until elastic. Divide into 8 equal portions; roll into balls, tucking in edges underneath to make dough look seamless. Using a rolling pin, flatten each out to roughly the size of skillet's cooking surface.

4. Set skillet over medium heat. Fry flatbreads one at a time until small pockets of air develop within; flip and continue cooking until lightly brown on both sides. Place cooked pieces on a serving platter lined with tea towel.

5. Using pastry brush, lightly grease both sides of the flatbread with oil. Cover platter with another tea towel to prevent bread from drying out. Repeat step until all flat breads are cooked.

6. Place 2 pieces on plates; slice these into wedges. Serve with desired amount of dipping sauce on the side.

Nutrition:

Protein 2.8g (5%), Potassium (K) 179 mg (4%), Sodium (Na) 135 mg (9%)

FRUITY CRUMBLE

———— ⚬⁓ ————

Preparation time: 10 minutes Cooking Time:30 minutes Servings: 6

INGREDIENTS:

- ½ cup unsalted butter
- 1 cup chopped rhubarb
- 1 cup all-purpose flour
- ½ cup brown sugar
- ½ tsp cinnamon
- 2 apples, peeled, cored, and thinly sliced
- 2 tbsps granulated sugar
- 2 tbsps water

DIRECTIONS:

Preheat an oven to 325ºF.Grease a 8x8-inch baking dish with some butter.

In a mixing bowl, add flour, sugar, and cinnamon. Combine to mix well with each other.

Add butter and combine well until your feel coarse crumbs.

Take a medium saucepan or skillet, add rhubarb, apple, sugar and water. Put over medium heat for 18-20 minutes until rhubarb is soft.

Pour over baking dish and add crumbs on top.

Bake for 20-30 minutes until golden brown.

Serve warm.

NUTRITION: Calories 443, Fat 21g, Phosphorus 61mg, Potassium 193mg, Sodium 28mg, Carbohydrates 54g, Protein 4g

LEMON COOKIES

Preparation time: 10 minutes Cooking Time: 10 minutes Servings: 2

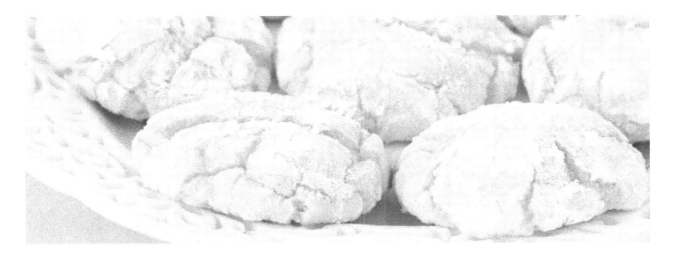

INGREDIENTS:

- 1 egg
- 1 ½ tsps lemon extract
- 1 ½ cups all-purpose flour, sifted
- 1 cup unsalted butter or margarine
- 1 cup granulated sugar

DIRECTIONS:

Preheat an oven to 375ºF.

In a mixing bowl, add butter and sugar. Combine to mix well with each other.

Beat an egg and add it with the mixture. Add lemon extract; beat until it is light and fluffy.

Add flour and mix until it becomes smooth.

Drop the batter by tbsp measure over an ungreased cookie sheet. Keep a 2-inch space between each drop.

Bake for about 10 minutes until turn evenly brown.

Serve warm.

NUTRITION:

Calories 138, Fat 5g, Phosphorus 31mg, Potassium 27mg, Sodium 19mg, Carbohydrates 13g, Protein 2g

BANANA PUDDING

Preparation time: 3 hours Cooking time: 0 minutes Servings: 12

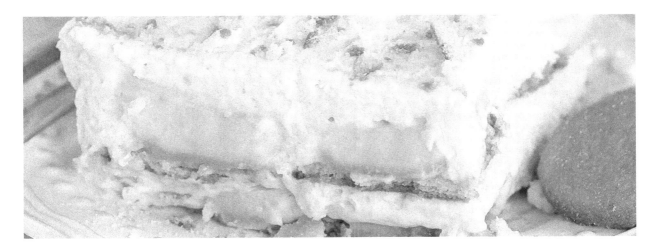

INGREDIENTS:

- 2 boxes Jell-O Cook and Serve banana cream pudding mix
- 12 ounces vanilla wafers
- 8 ounces dairy whipped topping
- 2½ cups unenriched rice milk

DIRECTIONS:

Line bottom of a 9x13-inch pan with vanilla wafers.

Mix 2 boxes of banana pudding mix with 2½ cups rice milk in a medium saucepan. Bring to a boil over medium heat. Keep stirring.

Pour pudding mixture over the vanilla wafers.

Place the second layer of vanilla wafers over first. Press each one down gently.

Refrigerate for 1 hour.

Keep in the refrigerator for 2 hours before serving.

NUTRITION:

Protein 3g, Carbohydrates 46g, Fat 7g, Calories 259

CHAPTER 9:
30 DAY MEAL PLAN TO REPAIR THE KIDNEYS NATURALLY

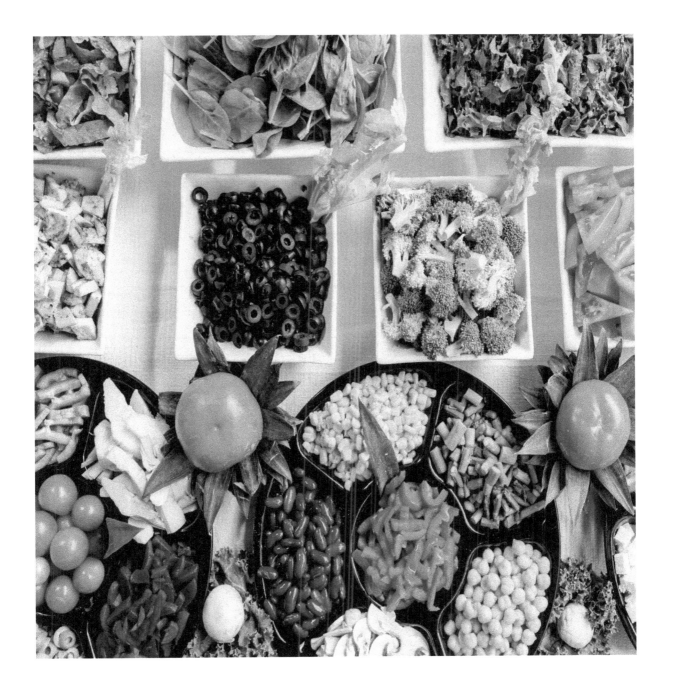

DAYS	BREAKFAST	LUNCH/DINNER	DESSERTS AND SNACKS
DAYS 1	Parmesan Zucchini Frittata	Beef Stroganoff Soup	Lemon Squares
DAYS 2	Texas Toast Casserole	Buffalo Ranch Chicken Soup	Creamy Pineapple Dessert
DAYS 3	Apple Cinnamon Rings	Paprika Pork Soup	Blackberry Mountain Pie
DAYS 4	Zucchini Bread	Coffee and Wine Beef Stew	Buttery Lemon Squares
DAYS 5	Garlic Mayo Bread	Beef Stew	Chocolate Gelatin Mousse
DAYS 6	Yogurt Bulgur	Bacon Cheeseburger Soup	Blackberry Cream Cheese Pie
DAYS 7	Chia Pudding	Pork Steaks	Almond Milk Coffee and Chocolate
DAYS 8	Goat Cheese Omelet	Pork and Veggie Skewers	Cashew Creamed Coffee with Cocoa Nibs
DAYS 9	Vanilla Scones	Pork with Bamboo Shoots and Cauliflower	Coconut Creamed Coffee with Cinnamon
DAYS 10	Olive Bread	Crispy Pork Shoulder	Pecan Pancake
DAYS 11	Yufka Pies	Frittata with Spicy Sausage	Almond Milk Coffee and Blueberry

DAYS 12	Breakfast Potato Latkes with Spinach	Pork Stir-Fry Chinese-Style with Muenster Cheese	Blueberry muffins
DAYS 13	Cherry Tomatoes and Feta Fritatta	Slow Cooker Hungarian Goulash	Oven Baked Eggplant Fries
DAYS 14	Egg White Scramble	Pork and Bell Pepper Quiche	Gluten-free Dark Choco Almond Butter
DAYS 15	Beet Smoothie	Grilled salsa	Mango Pear Salsa
DAYS 16	Cinnamon Apple Water	Ground Turkey with Veggies	Upland Cress and Cauliflower Open-Faced Sandwich
DAYS 17	Apple and Beet Juice Mix	Turkey & Pumpkin Chili	Zucchini Chips
DAYS 18	Protein Caramel Latte	Cranberry-lime apple spritzer	Carrot Muffin Cake
DAYS 19	Lime Spinach Smoothie	Chicken tortilla soup	Blueberry baked bread
DAYS 20	Protein Coconut Smoothie	Grilled Halloumi and Tuna Salad	Herb bread
DAYS 21	Strong Spinach and Hemp Smoothie	Tuna Fillets with Greens	Oatmeal Berry Muffins
DAYS 22	Total Almond Smoothie	One-Pot Seafood Stew	Berry Fruit Salad with Yogurt
DAYS 23	Ultimate Green Mix Smoothie	Easy Parmesan Crusted Tilapia	Ambrosia
DAYS 24	Chocolate Smoothie	Hearty Chicken Rice Combo	Apple Bars
DAYS 25	Orange Pineapple Shake	Homemade apple sauce	Egg Custard
DAYS 26	Fruit Vanilla Shake	Grilled Chicken	Chocolate & Coffee Mousse

DAYS 27	Almond Milk	Grilled Chicken with Pineapple & Veggies	Chocolaty Avocado Mousse
DAYS 28	Rosemary Watermelon Water	Mediterranean Burrito	Chocolaty Chia Pudding
DAYS 29	Parmesan Zucchini Frittata	Scallop Ceviche	Carrot Chia Pudding
DAYS 30	Texas Toast Casserole	Yeast dinner rolls	Apple Chia Pudding

CONCLUSION

——— ❧ ———

Kidney disease now ranks as the 18th deadliest condition in the world. In the United States alone, it is reported that over 600,000 Americans succumb to kidney failure.

These stats are alarming, which is why it is necessary to take proper care of your kidneys, starting with a kidney-friendly diet.

These recipes are ideal whether you have been diagnosed with a kidney problem or you want to prevent any kidney issues.

Taking care of your kidneys is vital to a healthy life. You have to provide a healthy environment for your kidneys to prevent further cell damage and possible kidney disease. A proper renal diet like the one explained in this cookbook can help you improve or maintain your kidney health by cutting down on the minerals that destabilize the internal balance of your kidneys: sodium, potassium and phosphorus.

In this cookbook, we tried to offer you the best possible renal diet recipes for everyday consumption ranging from breakfasts to side dishes, snacks, soups, salads, smoothies, meat and desserts.

The diet plays a key role in maintaining kidney health; in fact, the scraps of ALL the previously digested-absorbed-metabolized nutritional molecules are filtered by the circulatory stream thanks to the kidneys, then collected in the bladder and expelled with urine through urination.

Following a Renal Diet means following a diet that may be less taxing on your kidneys and therefore may slow the development of kidney disease.

A renal diet is tied in with directing the intake of protein and phosphorus in your eating routine. Restricting your sodium intake is likewise significant. By controlling these two variables you can control the vast majority of the toxins/waste made by your body and thus this enables your kidney to function at 100%. If you get this book early enough and truly moderate your diet with extraordinary consideration, you could avert an all-out renal failure. If you get this early, you can take out the issue completely.

Good luck.

RENAL DIET COOKBOOK

FOR VEGETARIAN & VEGAN

How to Repair the Kidneys Naturally. 79 Original and Healthy Recipes to Prevent Kidney Disease and Improve Your Physical Well-Being

BY MICHELLE BURNS

INTRODUCTION

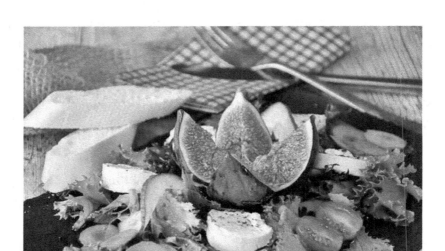

The fine cuisine for those who have to adhere to a: cholesterol-restricted, sodium-restricted, calorie-restricted, fat-restricted, fiber-restricted, fiber-rich, sugar-free or kidney diet and for people who love good food.

"This book contains a wide selection of recipes. These recipes makes it clear that healthy eating with certain restrictions does not necessarily mean that one should be deprived of all kinds of delicious food. Diets in particular follows a large number of recipes, from appetizers and soups to pies and desserts, always starting with a basic recipe, and then making adjustments for an energy (calorie) restricted diet, fat restricted diet, cellulose (fiber) enriched diet or restricted diet or kidney diet,

A renal diet is one that is low in phosphorous, protein, and sodium. The importance of eating high-quality protein and typically limiting fluids is often emphasized by a renal diet. Potassium and calcium may also need to be restricted in some patients. Every person's body is different, so it is important for each patient to work with a renal dietitian to establish a diet customized to the needs of the patient.

People who have kidney disease normally need to follow a minimal diet to help regulate chemical and fluid levels in their blood. This will make it difficult for you and your family to find delicious daily meals and recipes. This book helps to get the right balance between making the making the necessary changes to your diet and enjoying your food.

These combination options in this book makes it an excellent one for families, in which different diets have to be taken into account, or in which one diet is combined with a normal, but responsible menu. It is also a suitable cookbook for dietitians, cooks and housekeepers associated with an institution.

A cookbook for people who appreciate a good meal. Not only for those who have to, but also for those who want to spare themselves to stay healthy. "

CHAPTER 1: THE ROLE OF KIDNEYS IN OUR SYSTEMS?

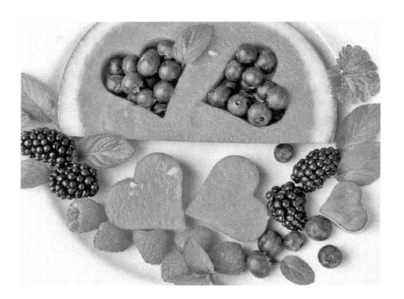

The kidneys are among the most essential organs of the human body. Kidney malfunctions can lead to severe illness or even death. Each kidney has a very complex function.

In particular, they have two essential functions: to flush out toxic and harmful waste products and maintain fluid, mineral, water, and chemical balance, i.e., electrolytes such as potassium, sodium, etc.

Structure of the Kidney

The kidney produces urine by eliminating excess water and toxic waste products from the body.

Urine formed in each kidney goes through the ureter, flows into the bladder before eventually excreted through the urethra.

Most people have two kidneys.

- The kidneys are situated at the top and back of the abdomen on either side of the spine. They are secured from damage by the lower ribs.
- The kidneys lie deep within the abdomen, so one can not feel them normally.
- The kidneys are a pair of bean-shaped organs. A kidney is about 10 cm long, 4 cm thick, and 6 cm wide in an adult. Each kidney weighs approximately 150-170 grams.

Urine produced in the kidneys flows down and then through the ureters to the urinary bladder. Each ureter is approximately 25 cm long and is a hollow tube-like structure consisting of special muscles.

The urinary bladder is a hollow organ made up of muscles that lie in the abdomen's lower and anterior parts. It acts as a urine reservoir.

The adult urinary bladder carries about 400-500 ml of urine; a person feels the urge to urinate when filled to near capacity.

During the urination process, the urine in the bladder is excreted by the urethra. The urethra is relatively short in females, whereas it is much longer in males.

Why are the kidneys essential for a living?

- Every day, we eat various types and quantities and kinds of food.
- The quantity of salts, water, and acids in our body also varies daily.
- The continuous process of transforming food into energy produces harmful toxic materials.
- These variables contribute to changes in the body's amount of electrolytes, acids, and electrolytes. It can be life-threatening to accumulate unnecessary toxic materials.
- The essential job of flushing out harmful and toxic by-products is carried out by the kidney. At the same time, they also maintain and regulate the right balance and levels of acids, water, and electrolyte.

What are the functions of the kidney?

The kidney's primary function is to produce urine and purify the blood. Each kidney eliminates waste materials and other chemicals that the body does not need. Below are the most important functions of the kidney.

Removal of waste products

- The most significant feature of the kidney is the purification of blood by eliminating waste materials.

- There is protein in the food that we consume. Protein is required for the growth and repair of the body. However, when protein is used by the body, it creates waste products. It is similar to storing poison within the body to accumulate and maintain these waste products. The blood and toxic waste products that are subsequently excreted in the urine are filtered by each kidney.

- Urea and creatinine are the two major waste products that can easily be measured in the blood. Their "values" in blood tests reflect the role of the kidney. The value of creatinine and urea in the blood test would be high if both kidneys fail.

Removal of excess fluid

- The kidney's second most important function is to regulate fluid balance by excreting excess water as urine while maintaining the required amount of water in the body, vital for living. As the kidneys fail, they lose the ability to eliminate this excess amount of water. Excess water in the body results in swelling.

Balance minerals and chemicals

- The kidneys play another important function of regulating minerals and chemicals like potassium, sodium, calcium, phosphorus, hydrogen, bicbonate, and magnesium and maintain the normal composition of body fluid.

- Changes in the level of sodium can affect the mental state of the person. In contrast, changes in potassium level can have significant adverse effects on heart rhythm and muscle functioning. Maintenance of a normal level of phosphorus and calcium is vital for healthy bones and teeth.

Control of blood pressure

- The kidneys contain various hormones (renin, aldosterone, angiotensin, prostaglandin, etc.) that help regulate the salt and water in the body, which play a significant role in maintaining good blood control pressure. Disturbances in hormone production and water regulation and salt in a patient with kidney failure can lead to high blood pressure.

Red blood cells production

- Another hormone produced in the kidneys is erythropoietin, which plays an important role in red blood cell production. Erythropoietin production is reduced during kidney failure, leading to decreased RBC production, resulting in low hemoglobin (anemia). This is why the hemoglobin count does not increase in patients with kidney failure, despite supplementation with iron and vitamin preparations.

To maintain healthy bones.

- The kidneys process vitamin D into its active form, which is essential for absorbing calcium from food, the growth of teeth and bones, and keeping the bones strong and healthy. Decreased active vitamin D during kidney failure leads to decreased and weakened bone growth. Growth retardation may be a sign of kidney failure in children.

How Is Blood Purified And Urine Formed?

The kidneys retain all required substances throughout the blood purification process and selectively extract excess fluid, electrolytes, and waste products. Let us understand this complicated and incredible urine forming process.

- Did you know that 1200 ml of blood enters the kidneys for purification every minute, which is 20 percent of the heart pumps' total blood? So, 1700 liters of blood will be purified in one day!
- This process of purification occurs in filtering units known as nephrons.
- Each kidney contains approximately one million nephrons, and each nephron is made up of tubules and glomerulus.
- Glomeruli are filters with very tiny pores that have a selective filtration function. They effectively filter water and small-sized substances through them. However, larger-sized white blood cells, red blood cells, protein, platelets, etc. cannot pass through these pores. Therefore, such cells are not usually seen in healthy people's urine.

The kidney's key function is the removal of waste, excess water, and harmful products in the form of urine.

- The initial phase of urine formation occurs in the glomeruli, where 125 ml of urine is filtered per minute. It is quite surprising that in 24 hours, 180 liters of urine is formed. It contains not only electrolytes, waste products, toxic substances, but glucose and other useful substances.

- Each kidney performs the process of reabsorption with great precision. Ninety-nine percent of the fluid is selectively reabsorbed from 180 liters of fluid that enters the tubules, and only the remaining 1 percent of the fluid is excreted as urine.
- All important substances and 178 liters of fluid are reabsorbed in the tubules through this intelligent and precise procedure, while 1-2 liters of fluids, waste products, and other harmful substances are excreted.
- Urine formed by the kidneys flows to the ureters, passes into the urinary bladder, and is gradually excreted by the urethra.

Can there be variation in the volume of urine in an individual with a healthy kidney?

- Yes. The amount of water intake and ambient temperature are significant factors that determine the amount of urine produced by a normal person
- Urine tends to be concentrated when water intake is low, and its volume is decreased, but when a large volume of water is consumed, more urine is formed.

During the summer months, the volume of urine decreases due to transpiration induced by high ambient temperatures. During winter months, it is the other way round – no perspiration, low temperature, and more urine.

If the amount of urine is less than 500 ml or more than 3000 ml in a person with a normal water intake, it might mean that the kidneys need closer attention and further examination.

CHAPTER 2: CHRONIC KIDNEY DISEASE

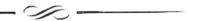

Chronic kidney disease involves conditions that damage your kidneys and reduce their ability to keep you healthy. If your kidney condition gets worse, waste will build up in your blood to high levels and make you feel sick. Complications such as high blood pressure, weak bones, poor nutritional health, anemia (low blood count), and nerve damage may develop. Also, kidney disease raises the risk of having heart and blood vessel disease. These issues can happen slowly over a long period of time. Diabetes, high blood pressure and other disorders can cause chronic kidney disease. Treatment and early diagnosis will also prevent chronic kidney disease from getting worse. It can ultimately lead to kidney failure as kidney disease progresses, requiring dialysis or a kidney transplant to sustain life.

The Facts About Chronic Kidney Disease (CKD)

- 37 million American adults have Chronic Kidney Disease and millions of others are at increased risk.
- Early detection can help prevent kidney disease from progressing to kidney failure.
- The main cause of death for all persons with CKD is heart disease.
- The best estimate of kidney function is the glomerular filtration rate (GFR).
- Hypertension triggers CKD and hypertension is caused by CKD.
- Persistent proteinuria (protein in urine) indicates CKD is present.
- High-risk categories include those with hypertension, diabetes , and family history of kidney failure.
- There is an increased risk for African Americans , Hispanics, Pacific Islanders, American Indians and seniors.
- CKD can be detected by two basic tests: blood pressure, serum creatinine and urine albumin.

What causes CKD?

Diabetes and high blood pressure are the two primary causes of chronic kidney disease. They are responsible for up to two-thirds of the cases. Diabetes occurs when your blood sugar is too high, causing damage to many of the body's organs, including the kidneys and heart, as well as blood vessels, eyes, and nerves. Hypertension, or high blood pressure, occurs when the pressure of your blood against the walls of your blood vessels increases. High blood pressure may be a leading cause of heart attacks, strokes and chronic kidney disease if uncontrolled, or poorly regulated. Also, chronic kidney disease can lead to high blood pressure.

Other conditions that affect the kidneys are:

- Glomerulonephritis, a group of illnesses that cause the filtering units of the kidney to be inflamed and impaired. These disorders are the third most common kind of kidney disease.
- Inherited diseases, such as polycystic kidney disease, cause the development of large cysts in the kidneys and destroy the tissue surrounding them.
- Malformations that occur when a baby grows in the womb of its mother. For instance, a narrowing may occur that prevents normal urine outflow and causes urine to flow back to the kidney. This causes infections and the kidneys can be damaged.
- Lupus and other diseases that affect the immune system of the body.
- Obstructions caused by disorders in men such as kidney stones, tumors or an enlarged prostate gland.
- Frequent urinary infections.

What are the symptoms of CKD?

Most individuals do not have any significant symptoms until their kidney disease is advanced. However, you may realize that you:

- have trouble concentrating
- feel more tired and have less energy
- have muscle cramping at night
- have a poor appetite
- have swollen feet and ankles
- have trouble sleeping

- have puffiness around your eyes, especially in the morning
- need to urinate more often, especially at night.
- have dry, itchy skin

Anyone can get chronic kidney disease at any age. Some individuals are, however, more likely to develop kidney disease than others. You could be at increased risk of developing kidney disease if you:

- have high blood pressure
- have diabetes
- are older
- have a family history of kidney failure
- belong to a population group that has high blood pressure or high rate of diabetes, such as Hispanic Americans, African Americans, Asian, American Indians, and Pacific Islanders.

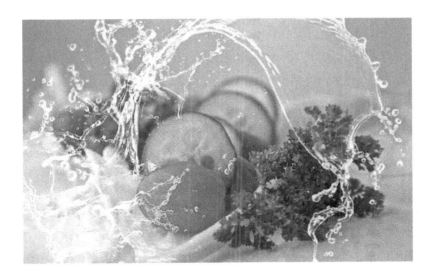

CHAPTER 3: SLOWING KIDNEY DISEASE

Having your kidneys function — even a little — can help you feel better and live longer. You will delay the need for treatment for kidney failure if you can slow your CKD. The kinds of improvements you might make to improve your heart, or your kidneys will also be helped by the rest of your body. Here are several things that you should do or avoid to protect your kidneys:

Blood sugar meter

Maintain the blood sugar within the target range. Blood vessels, including nephrons in the kidneys, are affected by high blood sugar. Your doctor will give you a target for fasting blood sugar if you have diabetes and for two hours after you eat. Test your blood sugar regularly to see how it changes depending on what you eat and how active you are. If you haven't done this yet, cut down on added sugar and processed carbs, such as bread, cakes, and rice. Take walks or find other ways to be active. Take your diabetes medicine(s) as prescribed.

- Maintain your blood pressure in the target range given to you by your doctor, too. Even if your blood pressure has been low throughout your life, it may now be high and it may be difficult to regulate. In CKD, it is common to require more than one drug for blood pressure. Check your blood pressure at home. Keep a log of the results so that you can tell your care team when it is high or low and what time you take your blood pressure pills. If you have side effects, speak with your doctor; a different medicine could work better for you. Exercise can also help reduce blood pressure.

- Lose Weight If You Are Overweight. The ten-year CARDIA study of young individuals (average age of 35) discovered that the more people weighed, the faster their kidney function decreased. This was true even though they did not have high blood pressure or diabetes. It's hard to lose weight, but it can be done, and it can work in a lot of ways. Ask for your care team's assistance if you need it.

- Don't drink soda. Drinking one or more sodas daily has been linked to kidney damage according to a large study. A second study discovered that two or more diet sodas a day can lead to kidney damage or make it progress faster.

- If you smoke or use street drugs, try to stop! Kidneys may be affected by smoking and most street drugs. If quitting was easy, of course, everybody would do it. There are a variety of ways to stop smoking, from going cold turkey to patches, e-cigarettes, or nicotine gum. Even cutting back may help. You may need a rehab program if you use street drugs. Talk to your care team if you need help to stop a habit that is affecting your health.

- Balance your blood pH. A healthy blood pH is between 7.38 and 7.42. When the kidneys don't function well, they will fail to maintain the acid-base balance in your body. Acid can build up from protein foods you eat. Grains and protein foods such as eggs, dairy, meat, beans, and peas form acid wastes then they break down. Your body requires protein for muscles and self–repair. Most of us, though, consume a lot more protein than we need. One way to make the kidneys last longer, at least if you are older, is to have a low-acid diet (with lots of veggies). Ask your doctor if you can help protect your kidneys with sodium bicarbonate, too.

Examples of dairy products

- Eat Less Protein. This forms blood urea nitrogen (BUN) as protein breaks down. It is difficult on the kidneys to extract BUN. You produce less BUN when you consume less protein, which can help your kidneys last a little longer. Research has shown that it may benefit much more to consume very little protein, but this is difficult to do and there is a risk of malnutrition.

- Eat Less Phosphorus. Phosphorus is present in meat, dairy, nuts, poultry, fish, beans, and cola drinks. Weak kidneys are unable to get as much phosphorus out of your blood. When your levels are too high, it can make your bones fragile.

- Limit Shellfish. Studies have shown that in mice, a toxin called domoic acid in shellfish and certain fish eating algae can damage the kidneys. People aren't mice. But, the really alarming result was that the kidneys could be affected by very small amounts of the toxin. Shellfish also have high purine levels, which, if you have gout, can be a concern. So, if you eat a lot, it might be prudent to cut back on shellfish.

- Skip Canned Foods. In the United States, most food cans are filled with bisphenol A (BPA). BPA has been associated with high blood pressure, diabetes, and obesity. Most packaged foods tend to have a very high salt or sugar content and are often highly processed. Glass jars or shelf safe cartons do not have BPA.

- Avoid Certain Pain Pills." Non–steroidal anti–inflammatory drugs" (NSAIDs) like Aleve®, Motrin®, and Advil® can cause kidney damage. Kidneys need a strong blood flow to function. NSAIDs minimize the flow of blood into and out of the kidneys. It takes years of everyday use for NSAIDs to cause CKD, in most cases. But NSAIDs will make it get worse faster, once CKD is present. Speak to your doctor about pain relief options that won't hurt your kidneys any further. If you take one tablet here and there and your kidneys are still functioning, drink a full glass of water with it.

- Need A Contrast Dye X – ray? Ask For Kidney Precautions. Dye that is injected into a vein for a CT or MRI scan will pass through your kidneys. Kidney damage may be caused by a dye called gadolinium. This dye can also cause an unusual problem called nephrogenic systemic fibrosis. NSF can be fatal, and can make the skin and organs thicken. There is no treatment for NSF. If a doctor orders an X-ray dye examination, ask if there are other ways to discover the same things. Would an ultrasound work, instead? Be sure to tell the radiologist about your CKD if you need to have a comparison. He or she might be able to dilute the dye or to wash it out of your blood by giving you an IV with sodium bicarbonate.

- Antioxidants May Help You. Every cell in the human body needs oxygen. But, excess oxygen in the wrong places can "oxidize" and cause damage, much like rust. Antioxidants may help your kidneys and it help protect your cells. Ask your doctor if antioxidants might be worth taking:

- Turmeric
- Coenzyme Q10

CKD is a risk factor for stroke and heart disease. The heart and blood vessels often appear to be affected by the same diseases that affect the kidneys. The good news is that moving gets your blood flowing, which boosts your kidneys' blood flow, and helps your heart. So, exercise is a win-win for your body. It can also help to slow the CKD rate.

The goal is thirty minutes of active movement daily. And, the thirty minutes don't have to be all at once. You can split your exercise into ten–minute blocks if you like.

Thinking of starting an exercise plan? If it is been a while since you were active, first speak with your doctor. Start slow, and build up distance, time, or weight slowly. Track your progress in order to see how you are doing. You can even set targets and reward yourself when you reach them.

Exercise doesn't have to be on a machine at a pricey gym. Here are some other alternatives you may think about, and you can come up with more:

- Walking is great exercise, and if you have a loved one as a companion, you get time together. You can enjoy an outdoor stroll if the weather is good and you live in a safe place. Or, a lot of people walk in malls or at indoor tracks so they do not miss out. A jog-walk will give you a more vigorous workout (trading off walking and jogging).

- Take Up a Sport. From tennis to badminton to bowling, you can spend time with others and improve your fitness at the same time if there's a team sport you like.

- Do a little work. Paint a wall or a fence. Get out and pull any weeds or cut the shrubs in the yard. Use a push mower to mow the grass. Vacuum a couple of rooms. You will get something done, be active, and feel good about yourself.

- Dance, Skate, Play! Moving is moving, whether you jump on a trampoline, paddle a canoe or take your partner out for a spin. Think of what you liked as a kid-it might give you some ideas of things to try.

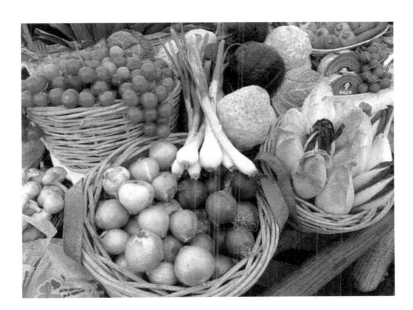

CHAPTER 4: NUTRITION AND CHRONIC KIDNEY DISEASE

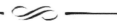

Understand your nutrient needs

Committing to a better eating habits is a good start. In order to understand how your diet affects your health. Let 's start with an overview of protein, carbohydrates, and fat, and why each is essential to maintain a healthy body when you have kidney disease.

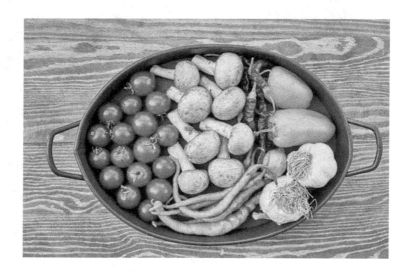

Carbohydrates

The bulk of your daily diet should be carbohydrates, since they are the body's primary source of nutrition. The body continually burns energy, even when at rest. The body requires energy not only for physical activities, but also for a variety of automatic functions, such as breathing and blood circulation. Without energy, your key organs cannot function.

Carbohydrates are categorized into two groups: simple and complex. Fruit is considered a simple carbohydrate and it is packed with energy, fiber and vitamins your body needs.

Complex carbohydrates are present in breads, grains and vegetables. These carbs provide vitamins and minerals as well as energy and fiber.

The goal is to choose sources of carbohydrates that do not "empty" calories, i.e. a carbohydrate food that has nutritional value. It is a waste of calories if a food doesn't have nutrients or vitamins that will sustain the body. People with diabetes can think about carbohydrates even more because regulating carbohydrate foods can help to control blood sugar levels.

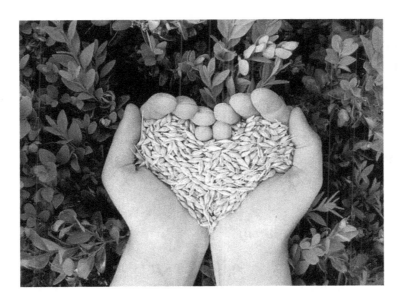

Protein

Protein develops muscle and repairs tissue. Protein is also used by the body to build antibodies, which are the anti-illness weapons of the body. Other chemicals in the body, such as enzymes and hormones, are produced from protein. Protein can mostly be found in animal sources (beef, pork, chicken, eggs , milk), but it can also be found in plant sources , especially soy products, nuts, and legumes. There are smaller quantities of protein in most vegetables, and fruit is practically free of protein.

Protein is vital for good health, however, in the later stages of chronic kidney disease, your doctor and renal dietitian can prescribe reducing the amount of protein you consume to reduce the stress on your kidneys as well as the accumulation of protein waste in the blood.

Fats

Fat is an essential component in our diets. It helps transport our cells with vitamins such as A, D , E and K. Fat is used to produce hormones such as estrogen and testosterone. Certain dietary fats that have fatty acids are healthy for our skin, make up linings of the body's cells and help with nerve transmission.However, too much fat can lead to weight gain, heart disease and other health issues.

Fats come in 2 categories: saturated and unsaturated. Saturated fats are present in dairy products and meat . These types of fats, particularly LDL (low density lipoprotein) cholesterol associated with heart disease and clogged arteries, may increase cholesterol. The FDA recommends that the number of saturated fats in your diet should be reduced. Unsaturated fats are present in nuts, fish, and specific oils. These types of fats can help reduce cholesterol. Food is often processed so that the unsaturated fat (such as soybean oil) is hydrogenated or partly hydrogenated. This process increases a type of fat *known as trans fatty acids.* Trans fat, like saturated fat, can increase the level of LDL and total cholesterol. For a balanced diet, the FDA advises the choice of foods low in both trans fats and saturated fats.

Potassium, sodium and phosphorus

These three minerals enable the body to function and the kidneys are carefully balanced. Some foods will need to be restricted as CKD progresses, since the kidneys can no longer get rid of excesses of these minerals taken in from the foods consumed. The doctor will order blood tests in order to track the levels of these minerals.

Nutrition for people with CKD

Proper nutrition is extremely essential for individuals with CKD. When blood pressure is elevated, a lower sodium diet can be recommended for patients in the early stages. Major changes in food consumption may not be the main focus of treatment. But this does not mean that you will not be able to take action to be as healthy as you can be. Food is the fuel that we bring into the body. A healthy diet allows our bodies to work effectively. Also, a healthy diet provides us with enough energy to support our level of activity. Too much food contributes to an excess of calories, which are processed as fat and leads to weight gain. Too little calories can lead to weight and loss of muscle.

Your doctor will refer you to a renal dietician if you are in the later stages. Your nutritionist will develop an eating plan to help you remain healthy and prolong the life of your kidneys.

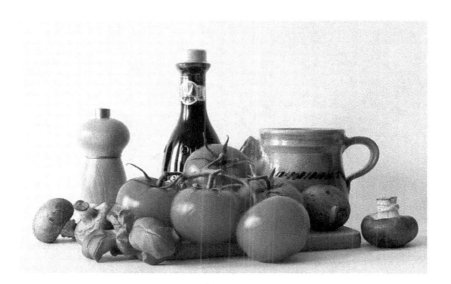

Chapter 5: Renal Diet Recipes

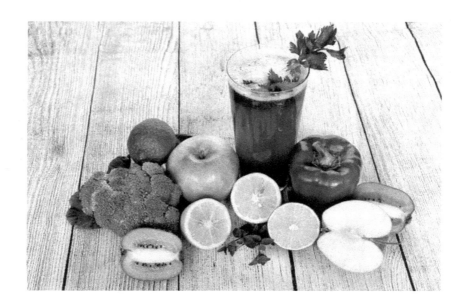

The dirty dozen list of fruits and vegetables

If you want to maximize the good you are doing for your body while minimizing costs, you can choose to buy organic fruits and vegetables that usually contain the most pesticides.

It is estimated that if a consumer eats non-organically grown products in the "dirty dozen" list, exposure to pesticides can be reduced by up to 80 percent.

This following list was compiled by the Environmental Working Group of approximately 96,000 USDA and FDA studies of the 49 fruits and vegetables listed between 2000 and 2015.

There are many fruits and vegetables that are not on this list - these are chosen because they are usually eaten.

- Celery (the worst)
- peaches
- strawberries

- Apples
- Blueberries (grown in the US)
- nectarines
- Sweet peppers
- Spinach
- Kale and collard greens
- cherries
- potatoes
- Grapes

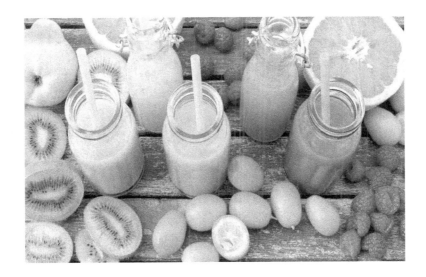

The Clean 15 It can be nice to buy non-organic

The "clean 15" is a list of products that are less likely to contain pesticides or are safer to buy conventionally because of the way it is eaten or protected from pesticides in the way it is grown or grown.

Clean 15 foods that are less likely to contain pesticides

- Avocado
- Sweet corn
- Pineapple
- Cabbage
- Sweet peas
- onions

- asparagus
- mangoes
- Papaya
- Kiwi
- Eggplant
- Grapefruit
- cantaloupe
- Cauliflower
- Sweet potatoes

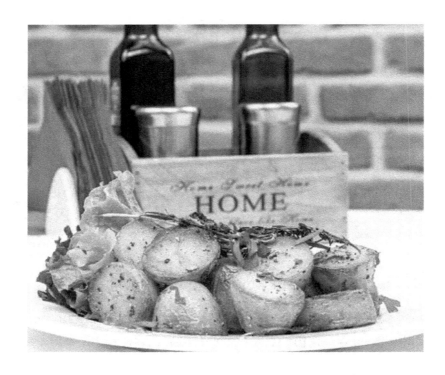

Kidney-potassium connection

People who have kidney problems should be careful about how much potassium they include in their diet. This is because the kidneys regulate potassium. If they do not work properly, potassium may not be expelled properly from the body.

To reduce potassium accumulation, a person with chronic kidney disease should follow a low-potassium diet between 1,500 and 2,000 milligrams (mg) per day. Limiting phosphorus, sodium and fluid can also be important for people with kidney dysfunction.

General rules

Torei Jones Armul, MS, RDN, CSSD, national spokesman for the Academy of Nutrition and Dietetics, offers several main rules:

- Avoid foods rich in potassium such as potatoes, bananas, whole grains, milk and tomato products.
- Watch out for portions of all foods.
- Watch your coffee. The National Kidney Foundation recommends people who should limit potassium to take coffee to one cup a day

There are many more nutritious, tasty options with little potassium for people with kidney disease, says Armul. These include berries, zucchini, corn, rice, poultry, fish and non-dairy substitutes.

Effective replacement

Beef and potato plate - the most important diet in the Midwest - contains a large amount of potassium. But another hearty meal, chicken and carrots, is much lower.

3 ounces of roast beef and half a cup of boiled potatoes would cost 575 mg of potassium. But one serving of chicken and carrots of the same size? This is less than 500 mg. Replacing carrots with boiled cauliflower, broccoli or asparagus also keeps you in that park.

Lots of fish in the sea

When it comes to fish, potassium levels drop along the entire line. You want to avoid surfing with high potassium intake, such as carrots, tuna, cod and fish. Portions of 3 oz can contain as much as 480 mg of potassium.

Below, the same amount of canned tuna has only 200 mg. Salmon, chicken, fish and pig produce about 300 mg per 3 oz meal.

Choices with low-potassium fruit

Vandana Sheth, RDN, CDE, a spokeswoman for the Academy of Nutrition and Dietetics, says that some fruits are ideal for those with a low-potassium diet.

An apple, the size of a tennis ball or a small or medium peach contains less than 200 mg of potassium, as well as half a cup of berries (blackberries, blueberries, raspberries, strawberries).

High-potassium fruits such as mangoes, bananas, papayas, pomegranates, prunes and raisins should be avoided.

Bananas are also full of potassium. Only one medium-sized banana contains 425 mg.

Selection of vegetables with low potassium

While vegetables usually contain a lot of potassium, Sheth says that there are many possibilities for fresh vegetables for those who need to watch their potassium levels. Vegetables containing less than 200 mg per meal include:

- asparagus (6 spears)
- broccoli (half a cup)
- carrot (cooked half a cup)
- corn (half ears)
- yellow zucchini or squash (half a cup)

Avoid potatoes, artichokes, beans, spinach, beet greens and tomatoes. Half a cup of dried beans or peas can contain as much as 470 mg of potassium.

Do not double the french fries

Sometimes people are forced to eat on the run. That's fine - just keep in mind how much potassium you're consuming. The American fast food product is a cheeseburger and french fries. The fast food cheeseburger contains between 225 and 400 mg of potassium.

One small serving of french fries? Huge 470 mg of potassium in just 3 oz. Just 1 oz of salted potato chips contains 465 mg.

Keep in mind what you drink

When it comes to drinks, milk contains a lot of potassium. One cup of milk can contain as much as 380 mg, while chocolate milk contains 420 mg.

Half a cup of tomato or vegetable juice contains about 275 mg of potassium, so you may be better off with orange juice, which contains only 240 mg.

Go easy on the sauce

Adding pasta and rice may not be something that many diet books recommend, but both are quite low in potassium. They contain between 30 and 50 mg per half cup. However, you need to be careful what you put on them. Just half a cup of tomato juice or tomato puree can contain as much as 550 mg of potassium.

Don't go too low

Just as it is important that people with kidney disease do not overdo it with potassium, so it should not be treated with potassium. Be sure to include at least some potassium in your diet. Fortunately, it is easy to get potassium in a generally balanced diet.

Potassium is an essential nutrient that we use to maintain the balance of fluids and electrolytes in the body, says Josh Ak, a certified nutritionist. It is needed for the function of several organs, including the heart, kidneys and brain. Talk to your doctor and dietitian about the right amount of potassium for you.

LET'S TALK ABOUT FOOD
Vitamins - Minerals - Probiotics – Laxatives

Due to the many restrictions in your diet, there may be a need for certain minerals and vitamins. Your doctor will prescribe the necessary supplements.

Never take supplements on your own initiative. They can contain minerals or vitamins that are harmful.

Probiotics (eg Yakult, Actimel) are used for a balanced and healthy intestinal flora but are rich in phosphorus.

Consult the dietitian.

In case of constipation:

- Never take fiber-rich supplements or herbal drinks (contain a lot of phosphorus and potassium)
- Before using laxatives, consult a doctor first
- Request the special brochure from the dietitian

Avoid constipation by:

Use gingerbread regularly

- Use sufficient fat on bread and in preparations
- On an empty stomach, take a spoonful of oil, possibly flavored with lemon juice
- Under no circumstances use supplemental amounts of vegetables, fruit or fiber (high in potassium)

Discussion of the foods

Fresh vegetables One portion of maximum 150 grams per day.

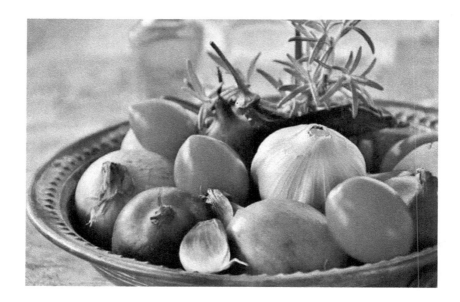

TIPS

- Clean the vegetables, cut them into small pieces and boil them in plenty of water.
- Never use the cooking liquid for preparing sauces.
- Finish the vegetables with a small amount of fat, onion, herbs and spices.
- White sauce can be used with vegetables, but do not do this too often.
- Never use tomato paste for the preparation of tomato sauce, but fresh tomatoes.
- This sauce can replace vegetables or potatoes. Replace potatoes with rice or pasta.
- The use of the microwave oven, steam oven, steam cooker, pressure cooker and wok should be avoided. These cooking techniques can only be used for heating up already blanched vegetables.
- Raw vegetables contain more potassium than prepared vegetables.

Potatoes, pasta, rice

Use a maximum of 150 grams potatoes per day. Replace the potatoes at least twice a week with white rice, pasta or couscous.

Peel the potatoes the day before, cut them into small pieces and leave them.

Boil the potatoes the day after in a generous amount of water.

Never use the cooking liquid from

French fries and baked potatoes can be used after the potatoes have first been blanched (soak in boiling water for two minutes and pat dry).

Potatoes.

- • Never cook the potatoes in a steamer, steam oven, microwave or pressure cooker.

Soup

Take your moisture restriction into account!

TIPS

- Soup is a source of extra potassium and moisture. Use the soup as a substitute for a hot meal along with bread and dessert, rather than before a meal.
- Be extra careful with soup on weekends and avoid soup if you gain too much weight between dialyses.

LIMITED USE TO AVOID

- Low-salt broth (= lean meat or chicken broth with herbs and no salt)
- Soup prepared on the basis of broth without salt (no stock cubes) and soup vegetables (without potatoes, legumes and tomato paste)
- Soup can optionally be combined with rice, vermicelli, tapioca. • Instant soup, frozen

soup; tin and cardboard

- Diet soup
- Tomato soup, mushroom soup, spinach soup and potato soup.
- Meat extract (eg Oxo), stock cubes
- If you use a meal soup (eg stew), prepare it without potatoes and use bread with it. The more vegetables in the soup, the more potassium. Do not add potatoes. Rice, pasta, tapioca and couscous are possible.
- If you use soup during the weekend, do not use fruit.

TIPS

- Canned fruit contains less potassium than fresh fruit. Never use the juice!
- One piece of fruit is the size of an apple (about 120 grams peeled).
- Always peel fruit.
- One glass of fruit juice = two to three pieces of fruit!

Meat, poultry, fish and meat substitutes It is important to consume meat, poultry or fish every day to ensure adequate protein intake in your diet. Regularly use fish (including fatty fish) and poultry instead of red meat. If you wish to use meat substitutes, first ask the dietician for advice. A vegetarian diet is difficult to combine with your diet!

TIPS

- Meat and fish can be prepared in the normal way.
- Preparations with tomatoes (e.g. balls in tomato sauce) are best prepared with fresh tomatoes and in this meal replace the vegetables or potatoes with rice, pasta or bread.
- Mussels contain a lot of phosphorus and potassium; use only half a kilo and use bread instead of fries.
- Fish and game contain more phosphorus than other meat; therefore, never use more than 150 grams per day.
- Be careful with crustaceans and shellfish: these are very rich in phosphorus and usually also very salty. So, reserve them for special occasions.

Eggs

Maximum two eggs per week to replace meat or fish: preparation method of your choice

(especially the yolk is rich in phosphorus)

Cheese

It is important to limit their use and to make the right choice. Solid cheeses, especially cheese spreads and processed cheeses, are extra rich in phosphorus and salt. Fresh, soft and semi-soft cheeses are therefore preferred. The low-fat variety of the cheeses (if it exists) is preferable to the fatty varieties.

In your daily menu, also take into account the cheese that you use in preparations.

Bread, cereals and thickeners
GOOD CHOICE

- White and light brown breads, white baguette, white pistolet, white piccolo
- Fantasy bread: milk bread, sugar bread, brioche bread, sandwich
- Coffee cakes: butter cake, croissant (without raisins and chocolate) gingerbread (without dried fruit)
- White rusks, toast, crispbread, Cracottes, rice cake
- Breakfast Cereals: Cornflakes, Frosties, Rice Krispies
- Binders: flour, potato starch, corn starch, wheat and rice semolina, pudding powder (vanilla, mocha)

AVOID THESE

- Whole wheat bread and multigrain bread, bran bread, rye bread,
- Fantasy bread with chocolate, dried fruit or nuts: raisin bread, chocolate bread, nut bread
- Coffee cakes with raisins, nuts and chocolate
- Whole wheat rusk and toast
- Whole grain cereals, cereals with dried fruits, nuts or chocolate
- Muesli, oatmeal
- Binders: chocolate pudding powder
- Fats, oils and savory sauce

GOOD CHOICE

- Oils: olive oil, corn oil, soybean oil, peanut oil, safflower oil, sunflower seed oil, nut oil, grape seed oil
- Margarine: Vitelma, Becel, Benecol
- Baking and frying fat: Becel baking and frying, Vitelma baking and frying, Becel liquid
- Frying oil: based on the permitted oils eg. Vitelma, Becel, Vandemoortele frying oil
- Sauce: vinaigrette and dressing: Becel dressing, yogonnaise
- Low-fat cream (light cream), soy cream (in moderation)

AVOID THESE

- Palm fat
- Coconut fat (used in biscuits, cakes and chocolate)
- Margarine,
- Butter, lard, herb butter, semi-skimmed butter
- Baking and frying
- Solid frying fat
- Ready-made sauce (too salty)
- Full cream
- All types of mayonnaise (also light mayonnaise and derived sauces, e.g. cocktail sauce). These sauces are made from egg yolks and are therefore a hidden source of phosphorus!
- Generous use of diet margarine on the bread and extra oil in the preparations provide the necessary calories.

Chapter 6: Vegetarian Dishes

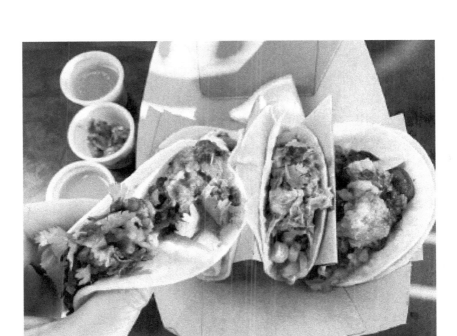

CAULIFLOWER CHEESE

This recipe uses cheese and milk which may mean that it is high in potassium and phosphate; however it makes a large amount of cauliflower cheese to serve four-six people. It should contain 25g/1oz of cheese and 125ml/ ¼ pt milk maximum per portion, which is within the allowances for those requiring restrictions.

Serves four-six

- One large cauliflower (leaves cut off), broken into pieces
- Four tbsp flour
- 500ml milk
- 100g (3½oz) strong cheddar, grated
- Two-Three tbsp breadcrumbs

- 50g (1¾oz) butter

Preparation method

1. Bring a big saucepan of water to the boil, add the cauliflower and cook for five minutes. Lift a slice to test, it should be cooked. Drain the cauliflower, then pour it into a dish that is ovenproof.
2. Heat the oven to 425 ° F / Gas 7 at 220 ° C (200 ° C fan).
3. Return the saucepan back to the heat and add the flour, butter, and milk. As the butter melts and the mixture comes to the boil, keep whisking quickly-the flour will vanish and the sauce will start thickening. Whisk for two minutes while the sauce bubbles and becomes smooth and thick. Turn the heat off, stir in much of the cheese and dump the cauliflower over it. Scatter over the remaining breadcrumbs and cheese.
4. In the oven, bake the cauliflower cheese for twenty minutes until it bubbles.

Tip: Make enough for six servings, even if you need less as spare portions can be frozen before being baked.

PUMPKIN RISOTTO

This is a filling meal, and while it contains butternut squash (a vegetable with moderate levels of potassium), it is made with rice (rather than potatoes), which decreases the potassium content of the dish. The cheese used for this recipe is minimal, but you can enjoy this meal without cheese, reducing the phosphate and fat content. Serves 3-4

- 570ml (one pint) vegetable such as low chicken stock or salt Bouillon
- One small onion, chopped
- Twelve fresh sage leaves, chopped finely
- Two tbsp olive oil
- Freshly ground black pepper
- 250g (9oz) pumpkin or butternut squash, diced small ● 50g (2oz) butter
- 170g (6oz) Arborio (risotto) rice
- Piece of vegetarian parmesan-style grating cheese or fresh parmesan (this is optional)

Preparation method

1. Heat the stock and simmer over a very low heat until almost boiling. Sweat the onion in the oil in a separate heavy-based saucepan until soft but not browned. A dd the chopped sage and cook.

2. To cover the grains with oil, add the rice and mix well for a few seconds, then pour one-third of the stock in and bring it to a gentle simmer. Cook until it absorbs nearly all the stock. Add the squash or pumpkin and a little more stock, and cook gently until the stock is absorbed.

3. Add the remaining stock until the pumpkin is soft and the rice al dente is sweet. You do not need all the stock, but it should be loose and creamy in texture.

4. Stir the butter into the risotto and add salt and pepper and season well.

5. Add the grated cheese and divide into four servings.

PASTRY-LESS QUICHE

This is a very flexible recipe, since rather than the tomatoes, peppers, and mushrooms you can easily substitute all of the vegetables with any of your favorite vegetables, such as peas and dried mint or squash and sage. This dish can be eaten hot or cold as well, making it perfect for home dinner or for a packed lunch. Note that both mushrooms and tomatoes are high potassium foods, but ok when consumed in small amounts.

Serves 4

- One green pepper, diced
- One red pepper, diced
- One onion, chopped
- 75ml milk
- 50g (1¾oz) grated cheddar cheese or use a lower phosphate cheese such as feta
- Eight medium mushrooms, sliced
- 250g (9oz) fat free natural cottage cheese
- Two large or Three medium tomatoes, sliced
- Five eggs

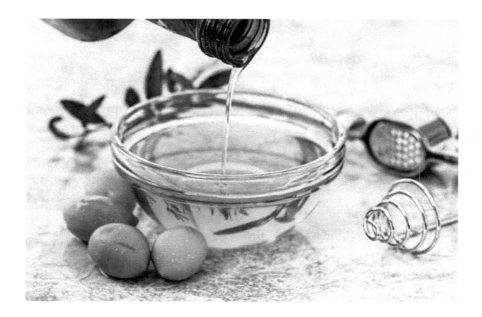

Preparation method

1. Using a small amount of vegetable oil or spray oil to gently fry prepared vegetables (except tomatoes). You still want to make them a little crunchy, so don't overdo the veg.
2. Mix the 5 eggs, 250 g fat-free natural cottage cheese and the milk together-this is not a pretty combination, but stick with it.
3. In an oven-proof flan dish, spread the chopped vegetables out, then pour over the cottage cheese mix.
4. Place the sliced tomatoes on top and sprinkle the cheese on top.
5. Pop in the oven at 190 ° C (170 ° C fan)/375 ° F / Gas 5, for about thirty to forty-five minutes, or until the quiche is golden brown.

TRADITIONAL COOKED ENGLISH BREAKFAST

Due to the high phosphate and potassium products it contains, many people avoid a typical cooked breakfast, but a cooked breakfast can still be enjoyed occasionally by complying with these guidelines.

Serves one

- One egg – any way you like
- Two pieces of bacon or one sausage (opt for low fat or remove fat if trying to lose weight)
- Four small mushrooms or one small tomato or two tbsp of baked beans
- As much toast as you like (however, be careful if you want to lose weight)

Preparation method

1. Grilling is the ideal cooking method if you are trying to lose weight, or you can fry with minimal oil in a non-stick frying pan or use spray oil.
2. Frying in fat will help increase the calories of your breakfast If you need to gain weight then.

HIGH ENERGY PORRIDGE

If you are underweight or accidentally lose weight, this high energy recipe is useful because it contains loads of extra calories.

Remember – if you are on a phosphate or fluid restriction then the milk should be excluded from your daily allowance for milk and fluid.

Serves One

- 35g (1¼oz) porridge oats
- 200ml full fat milk
- Optional: add cream and syrup or jam for extra energy

Preparation method

1. Mix all ingredients in a pan, heat the pan and boil for three to four minute.
2. Alternatively cook in the microwave for around one to two minutes, stirring at thirty second intervals.

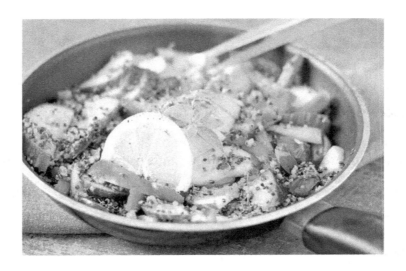

CRAB AND EGG BREAD
Nutritional values

Energy 150 kcal, Protein 6 g, BE 1, Carbohydrates 13 g, Potassium 150 mg, Phosphorus 90 mg

Ingredients for 1 serving

- 25 g Wheat toast bread (1 slice)
- 10 g Salad mayonnaise
- 10 g Lettuce
- 50 g Asparagus tips, canned food
- 10 g Egg slices (hard-boiled)
- 10 g Shrimp

To garnish:

- 1 g Sprig of dill
- 1 kl. Lemon wedge

Method

Toast the bread lightly and let it cool down.

Brush with mayonnaise and top with lettuce, asparagus, egg slices and shrimp.

Garnish with dill and lemon wedge.

POTATO SALAD
Nutritional values

Energy 319.2 kcal / Protein 5.8 g / P (phosphorus) 141.9 mg / K (potassium) 925.5 mg / Na (sodium) 154.1 mg

Ingredients

- potatoes 150 g
- onion 10 g
- apple 50 g
- celery 20 g
- carrot 10 g
- pickle 10 g
- eggs 15 g
- oil 15 g
- parsley, horseradish, vinegar, pepper, a pinch of salt

Method

Boil the whole potatoes in their skins. After cooling, peel and cut into cubes. Clean the celery, carrots and onions, grate finely. Boil the onions with hot water. We mix everything. Add grated apple, pickles, parsley, horseradish. Drizzle with oil, mix and leave to rest.

POTATO PANCAKES
Nutritional values

Energy 488.9 kcal / Protein 9.9 g / P (phosphorus) 198.9 mg / K (potassium) 1 189.2 mg / Na (sodium) 460.6 mg

Ingredients

- potatoes 250 g
- eggs 20 g
- flour hl 20 g
- oil 20 g
- pepper
- rubbed garlic
- marjoram
- pinch of salt

Method

Finely grate the raw washed and peeled potatoes. Drain excess water and add spices, flour, eggs. We will make the dough. Make small patties from the dough and bake in hot oil. A mixed salad with cheese goes well with potato pancakes.

CITRUS SALAD WITH SOUR CREAM
Nutritional values

Energy 76.8 kcal / Protein 1.5 g / P (phosphorus) 22 mg / K (potassium) 197.2 mg / Na (sodium) 81 mg

Ingredients

- grapefruit 50 g
- orange 50 g
- sour cream 25ml
- lemon juice
- salt

Method

Peel the grapefruit and oranges and remove the inner hard skins or kernels from them. Cut the fruit pulp into pieces, drizzle with lemon juice, lightly salt and pour over the cream.

TOASTS WITH TOMATOES AND TUNA
Nutritional values

Energy 399.6 kcal / Protein 9.3 g / P (phosphorus) 106.2 mg / K (potassium) 376.6 mg / Na (sodium) 186.9 mg

Ingredients

- White bread (low protein) 100 g
- tuna in a can 30 g
- tomatoes 100 g
- garlic 2 g
- fresh basil 5 g (1 teaspoon)
- olive oil 5 ml (1 teaspoon)
- mayonnaise (80% fat) 10 g
- lemon juice 5 ml (1 teaspoon)
- Worcestershire sauce 2 ml (½ teaspoon)

Method

Cut the bread or baguette into slices, which we bake. Boil the tomatoes, peel them, remove the grains and cut them into small pieces. Mix them with olive oil, garlic and basil. We mix tuna, mayonnaise, lemon juice, pepper and Worcester sauce separately. First, add the tomatoes and the tuna mixture to the toasted sandwiches and garnish with basil leaves.

MASHED POTATOES WITH CREAM
Nutritional values

Energy 226.9 kcal / Protein 3.7 g / P (phosphorus) 105.9 mg / K (potassium) 653.8 mg / Na (sodium) 493.8 mg

Ingredients

- boiled potatoes 150 g
- butter 10 g
- cream 10 g
- parsley

Method

Wash the potatoes, peel them, cut them and cook them soft. Drain the water from them and crumple. Add butter and warm cream to the mashed potatoes. Mix everything with a whisk into a fine slurry. Garnish on a plate with parsley.

RICE SOUP
Nutritional values

Energy 318.6 kcal / Protein 13.4 g / P (phosphorus) 32 mg / K (potassium) 160 mg / Na (sodium) 47.5 mg

Ingredients

- root vegetables 50 g
- rice 10 g
- butter 5 g
- vegetable broth
- parsley, pepper

Method

Fry the grated vegetables in butter and pour the broth. Add rice to the base and cook. Season the finished soup and garnish with parsley.

PEAR STUFFED WITH RICOTTA
Nutritional values

Energy 186.2 kcal / Protein 5.6 g / P (phosphorus) 112.7 mg / K (potassium) 293.1 mg / Na (sodium) 33.7 mg

Ingredients

- pear 160 g
- ricotta 30 g
- walnut 10 g
- lemon juice
- pepper
- chive

Method

First we prepare cheese cream = mix ricotta with pepper, lemon juice and grated nuts. Then we cut the pear in half and get rid of the core. Fill with cream. Serve with low-protein bread smeared with fat and decorated with chives.

GARLIC SPREAD
Nutritional values

Energy 173.8 kcal / Protein 8.9 g / P (phosphorus) 221.9 mg / K (potassium) 90.5 mg / Na (sodium) 462.6 mg

Ingredients

- garlic according to your own taste
- fresh cheese 50 g
- cottage cheese 20 g
- capsicum pepper 60 g
- chive
- salt

Method

Mix the grass and cottage cheese with crushed garlic, salt and chives. We spread on bread and decorate with peppers.

CELERY SPREAD
Nutritional values

Energy 293 kcal / Protein 14 g / P (phosphorus) 204 mg / K (potassium) 328 mg / Na (sodium) 358 mg

Ingredients

- celery 100 g
- lučina 50 g
- mayonnaise 10 g
- eidam 30 g

Method

We clean the celery and finely grate it. Mix with meadow grass, mayonnaise and grated cheese.

MIXED SALAD WITH CHEESE
Nutritional values

Energy 98.8 kcal / Protein 6.2 g / P (phosphorus) 120.7 mg / K (potassium) 404.4 mg / Na (sodium) 139.8 mg

Ingredients

- tomatoes 70 g
- cucumber sal. 50 g
- green pepper 50 g
- eidam cheese 15 g
- sugar 2 g
- oil 3 g
- vinegar

Method

Wash the tomatoes and cut into marigolds. Wash the pepper, remove the kernels and cut into strips. Wash the cucumber, peel and cut into slices. Drizzle with oil and pour over the dressing. We prepare the dressing from water, where we let the sugar and vinegar dissolve. Let it rest for about 1 hour and decorate with grated cheese. Eidam cheese can be exchanged for fresh cheese with dill.

SPAGHETTI WITH TOMATO SALSA
Nutritional values

Energy 467.1 kcal / Protein 12.8 g / P (phosphorus) 209.3 mg / K (potassium) 546.6 mg / Na (sodium) 43.2 mg

Ingredients

- spaghetti 100 g
- tomatoes 40 g

- onion 5 g
- garlic 2 g
- cream (30% fat) 20 ml
- fresh parsley 5 g
- fresh basil 5 g
- celery stem 2 g
- pepper ¼ g (1 pinch)

Method

Boil the tomatoes briefly with hot water and peel. Remove the grains from them and pour off the liquid, mix the pulp thoroughly. Fry the chopped onion, pepper, garlic (whole cloves) and parsley on part of the oil. Remove the garlic, add the tomato salsa and the rest of the oil. Simmer everything in the pot for about 10 minutes. Mix with pasta and serve.

BAKED CREAMY POTATOES
Nutritional values

Energy 353.7 kcal / Protein 11.7 g / P (phosphorus) 281.5 mg / K (potassium) 783.5 mg / Na (sodium) 178.3 mg

Ingredients

- potatoes 150 g
- onion 15 g
- plain flour 5 g
- sour cream 30 g
- fat 10 g
- parmesan 20 g

For broth:

- bay leaf, onion, thyme, fresh spices, pepper

Method

Peel the potatoes, cut into slices and cook. Put the spices in a pot, add water and cook the broth. We prepare a light dish from onion and oil and flour. Dilute the finished dish lightly with the broth and add the sour cream. We place boiled potatoes in a cleared form, which we pour with a dish. Pour grated cheese on the potatoes and bake until golden.

MASHED POTATOES
Nutritional values

Energy 271.7 kcal / Protein 6.1 g / P (phosphorus) 164.7 mg / K (potassium) 998.7 mg / Na (sodium) 68.8 mg

Ingredients

- Potatoes 200 g
- milk 60 ml
- butter 10 g

Method

Peel the potatoes, wash and cut. Put in a pot of cold water and cook until soft. Then drain the water and mash the potatoes. Add warm milk and whisk into a fine porridge. We can soften with a little butter.

BEETROOT RISOTTO
Nutritional values

Energy 641.4 kcal / Protein 12 g / P (phosphorus) 184.7 mg / K (potassium) 122.5 mg / Na (sodium) 77.7 mg

Ingredients

- rice 80 g

- onion 10 g
- cream (30% fat) 30 ml (3 tbsp)
- parmesan (40% fat) 10 g
- butter 20 g (4 teaspoons)
- beetroot juice 200 ml
- water 30 ml
- pepper ¼ g (1 pinch)
- nutmeg ¼ g (1 pinch)

Method

Fry the chopped onion in butter. After a few minutes, add the rice and stir until glassy. Add water and beetroot juice. We cook everything for 15-20 minutes. Season with salt, pepper and nutmeg and stir in the cream. Sprinkle with Parmesan cheese on a plate and serve.

BUBLANINA WITH COMPOTE FRUIT
Nutritional values

Energy 729.7 kcal / Protein 7.4 g / P (phosphorus) 132.2 mg / K (potassium) 78.9 mg / Na (sodium) 1 255 mg

Ingredients

- low-protein flour 6 g
- compote without juice 70 g
- eggs 1 pc
- sugar 25 g
- vanilla sugar 1 sachet
- baking powder
- solamyl 60 g
- fat 5 g
- oil 25 g
- water 1 tbsp

Method

Grease the mold and sprinkle with low-protein flour. In a side dish, whisk the egg yolk with the sugar into a foam. In another container, we whip snow out of the protein. Add oil and lukewarm water to the whipped foam and mix. We add solamyl, vanilla sugar and baking powder to the mass. Finally, lightly mix in the whipped snow. Pour the dough into a mold and add pieces of compote fruit without juice. Bake for 20-25 minutes. After baking, tilt and let cool.

TROUT CREAM ON WHITE BREAD
Nutritional values per serving:

Energy 260 kcal, Protein 9 g, Potassium 110 mg, Phosphorus 130 mg

Ingredients for 6 servings:

- 1 smoked trout
- 150 g creme fraiche Cheese
- 4 tbsp sour cream
- Pepper
- White bread

Method

The smoked trout, boning and peeling.

Cut the trout meat into small pieces, mash with a fork and mix with the creme fraiche and sour cream and season with ground pepper.

Simply spread the smoked trout cream on white bread and sprinkle with chives.

RICE PORRIDGE WITH STRAWBERRIES
Nutritional values

Energy 157.1 kcal / Protein 2.5 g / P (phosphorus) 61.5 mg / K (potassium) 187.8 mg / Na (sodium) 10.7 mg

Ingredients

- rice 20 g
- strawberries 100 g
- cream (20% fat) 10 ml
- sugar 10 g

Method

Rinse the rice and cook in lightly salted water until soft. When the rice is cooked, drain the excess water. Put the rice in bowls, sprinkle with strawberries, pour cream and sugar cane.

VEGETABLE FONDUE
Nutritional values

Energy 300 kcal / Protein 2 g / P (phosphorus) 59 mg / K (potassium) 430 mg / Na (sodium) 10.5 mg

Ingredients

- eggplant 50 g
- green pepper 50 g
- onion 25 g
- tomatoes 50 g
- olive oil 30 ml
- wine vinegar 10 ml
- pepper 1 g

Method

Cut the eggplant into thin slices. Salt them and let them sweat for a while, wash the liquid with water and dry the eggplants. Remove the stem and grains from the peppers and cut them lengthwise into 4 equal parts. Peel an onion and cut into thin slices. Boil the tomatoes, remove the skin and cut in half. Lightly rub oil in a large baking dish or baking dish and place the vegetables there. Pepper to taste and drizzle with 3 tablespoons of oil. Bake at 200 ° C for 35 min. After baking, remove the bowl from the oven and let it cool completely, then put it in the fridge. A few minutes before serving, we can drizzle the vegetables with a vinaigrette dressing, prepared from olive oil, lemon juice, wine vinegar, mustard, pepper and salt.

LOW-PROTEIN RUBBED SANDWICH
Nutritional values

Energy 1,074 kcal / Protein 4.2 g / P (phosphorus) 78.8 mg / K (potassium) 53.1 mg / Na (sodium) 51.6 mg

Ingredients

- solamyl 125 g
- vanilla pudding 40 g
- eggs 2.5 pcs
- sugar 100 g
- baking powder 1/4 pc
- oil 100 g
- vegetable fat (clearing the mold) 10 g
- solamyl (for emptying the mold) 30 g
- water 1 tbsp

Method

Grease the bread mold and sprinkle with solamyl. Beat the eggs with sugar and water into a foam. Mix oil and loose raw materials into the mixture. Pour the finished dough into a greased mold and bake for 25 minutes. After baking, tip the sandwiches and let them cool down. We can decorate the sandwich with hot raspberries or a scoop of whipped cream.

TUNA SALAD WITH PASTA
Nutritional values

Energy 782.2 kcal / Protein 26.5 g / P (phosphorus) 505 mg / K (potassium) 665.6 mg / Na (sodium) 457 mg

Ingredients

- low protein pasta 200 g
- tuna in its own juice 80 g
- tomato 50 g
- cucumber salad 50 g
- arugula 10 g
- mayonnaise 20 g

Method

We mix cooked pasta with cleaned and chopped vegetables and tuna. Add mayonnaise and stir.

PICNIC ROLLS

Nutritional values per serving

Energy 410 kcal, Protein 15 g, BE 3.5, Potassium 300 mg, Phosphorus 180 mg

Ingredients for 1 serving:

- 80 g Baguette rolls
- 15 g Diet or reform margarine
- 15 g Lettuce
- 25 g hard-boiled egg (½ pc, size M)
- 20 g boiled ham

- 10 g Radishes (1 pc.)
- 20 g red pepper, raw
- 3 g chives

Method

Cut open the roll and brush the inside with margarine.

Cut the egg and radishes into slices and cover the bread roll in colored order.

Cut the chives into fine rolls, sprinkle them on top of the bread and fold over the second half of the roll.

PESTO CREAM VEGGIE DIP

This dip recipe is perfect as a small meal, a dip to share with friends, or as a snack. Using cream cheese makes it low in phosphate and if served with crackers, corn crisps, or toasted pitta bread, instead than potato crisps they would be low in potassium too.

- 100g (3½oz) cream cheese
- 200g (7oz) basil pesto
- Two tablespoons parmesan cheese
- 100g (3½oz) sour cream

Preparation method

1. Place cream cheese, sour cream, pesto and parmesan cheese in a bowl and stir well.
2. Stir until chill and creamy. Ready to serve.

HEALTHY PORRIDGE

This porridge can be a healthy choice if you are ready to lose weight, since it is low in calories and high in fiber, which will make you stay full for longer, so you are less likely to snack before lunch. You may want to try rice or soya milk to supplement the skimmed milk if you are on a phosphate restriction since it is naturally lower in phosphate as well as low in fat.

Serves 1

- 100ml skimmed milk
- 35g (1¼oz) porridge oats
- Sprinkle of cinnamon
- ½ grated apple
- 100ml water

Preparation method

1. Mix all ingredients in a pan, heat the pan and boil for three to four minutes.
2. Alternatively cook in the microwave for around one to two minutes, stirring at thirty second intervals.

SOUPS, SNACKS, AND STARTERS
Goat's Cheese Rarebit

Do not be put off by the use of goat's cheese and soya milk in this recipe – they're both much lower in phosphate than cheddar and cow's milks and are equally tasty.

Serves two-four

- 25g (¾oz) flour
- 25g (¾oz) olive oil, butter or vegetable spread
- 175g (6oz) soft goat's cheese
- Four slices bread
- 150ml soya milk (we used unsweetened)
- Two egg yolks
- ½ tsp mustard
- Pepper

Preparation method

1. Place the butter or spread, cheese and soya milk in a saucepan and heat until melted

and smooth.

2. Stir in the flour, then bring the mixture to a boil, stir continuously while it thickens, .

3. Remove from the heat and add the pepper and mustard. Leave for five minutes to cool, then mix in the egg yolks with a fork.

4. Toast the bread on one side, turn over and split the rarebit blend between the slices.

5. Put under a hot grill and cook until golden and bubbling.

PLAIN SCONES

This is a staple recipe that is low in phosphate and potassium and works well as a snack, a pudding, or mall meal. It might sound a lot to make twelve in one go, but they freeze incredibly well-just make sure you use them within one month.

Makes 8-12

- 225g (8oz) self-raising flour
- 150ml milk
- 55g (2oz) butter
- One free-range egg, beaten, to glaze (use a little milk as an alternative)
- 25g (1oz) caster sugar
- pinch of salt

Preparation method

1. Heat the oven to 220°C (200°C Fan)/425°F/Gas 7. Grease a baking sheet lightly.

2. Mix the flour and salt together and rub in the butter.

3. Stir in the sugar, then the milk to get a soft dough.

4. Switch on to a work surface that is floured and knead very gently. Pat it out to a round 2cm/¾in thick. To stamp out rounds, use a 5 cm/2 in cutter and put them on a baking sheet. Lightly knead the remaining dough together and stamp out more scones to use it all up.

5. Use the beaten egg to brush the tops of the scones. Bake until well risen and golden.

SMOKED MACKEREL PATÉ

Enjoy this low phosphate paté on Melba toast, toasted bread, or any other cracker, if you're trying to lose weight then go for the low fat cream cheese.

Serves One-Six

- Two spring onions, trimmed and finely sliced
- 200g (7oz) smoked mackerel fillets, skin removed
- One lemon
- One tablespoon creamed horseradish
- Pepper
- 100g (3½oz) cream cheese

Preparation method

1. Break the mackerel into chunks and cut it finely.
2. Add the mackerel, spring onions, cream cheese, creamed horseradish and one lemon zest to a bowl and mix.
3. Squeeze your zested lemon juice into it, and mix again until the paste is coarse.
4. Season with pepper to taste.

CORN SALAD
Nutritional values

Energy 149.8 kcal / Protein 3.4 g / P (phosphorus) 105 mg / K (potassium) 307.6 mg / Na (sodium) 415.7 mg

Ingredients

- frozen corn 100 g
- yolk 1/4
- mustard 1/4 tablespoon
- oil 5 ml
- lemon juice

- sugar 5 g
- chive
- salt

Method

Boil frozen corn in salted water. Drain and allow to cool. Mix oil, lemon juice, sugar, mustard and egg yolk and pour over the corn. Garnish the salad with chopped chives.

QUICK AND EASY PANCAKES

This really is a simple recipe and can be topped with your choice of either savoury or sweet foods.

Serves 2-4

- One egg
- One cup* of milk
- Cooking oil or butter
- One cup* of flour (any type)

* cup = approximately 200ml

Preparation method

1. Place the milk, flour, and egg into a bowl and whisk to mix thoroughly to form a smooth batter.
2. Heat your frying pan until hot, add the butter or sunflower oil and a large spoonful of the pancake mix.
3. Fry over a medium heat for 10 to 15 minutes until golden brown underneath.
4. Turn the pancake over and cook for a further one-two minutes, or until it is cooked and golden brown.
5. Set this aside and repeat with the remaining batter.

Serving suggestions

Try with tinned pears or stewed apples, peaches, raspberries or strawberries and serve with single cream (remember that tinned fruit is lower in potassium than fresh).

Try serving topped with grated cheese or tuna, ham, or perhaps a hot filling such as chilli for a savoury pancake.

STUFFED EGGS WITH WILD GARLIC CREAM
Nutritional values per serving

Energy 190 kcal Protein 12 g BE 0.2 Potassium 170 mg Phosphorus 130 mg

Ingredients for 6 servings:

- 100 g Double cream cream cheese
- 250 g Lowfat quark
- 100 g creme fraiche Cheese
- Bunch of wild garlic
- 1 teaspoon Lemon juice
- pepper
- 6 hard-boiled eggs
- 6 radish
- Lettuce leaves for decoration

Method

Mix the cream cheese with the quark, creme fraiche and lemon juice until creamy.

Season with pepper and a little salt. Cut the wild garlic very finely and mix with the cream. Peel the eggs and carefully remove the yolks (do not process them further).

Fill the wild garlic cream into a piping bag with a large perforated nozzle and fill the hard-boiled egg halves.

Line a plate with lettuce leaves, place the filled eggs on top and garnish with radish slices.

CAULIFLOWER CHEESE

This recipe uses cheese and milk which may mean that it is high in potassium and phosphate; however it makes a large amount of cauliflower cheese to serve four-six people. It should contain 25g/1oz of cheese and 125ml/ ¼ pt milk maximum per portion, which is within the allowances for those requiring restrictions.

Serves four-six

- One large cauliflower (leaves cut off), broken into pieces
- Four tbsp flour
- 500ml milk
- 100g (3½oz) strong cheddar, grated
- Two-Three tbsp breadcrumbs
- 50g (1¾oz) butter

Preparation method

1. Bring a big saucepan of water to the boil, add the cauliflower and cook for five minutes. Lift a slice to test, it should be cooked. Drain the cauliflower, then pour it into a dish that is ovenproof.
2. Heat the oven to 425 ° F / Gas 7 at 220 ° C (200 ° C fan).
3. Return the saucepan back to the heat and add the flour, butter, and milk. As the butter melts and the mixture comes to the boil, keep whisking quickly-the flour will vanish and the sauce will start thickening. Whisk for two minutes while the sauce bubbles and becomes smooth and thick. Turn the heat off, stir in much of the cheese and dump the cauliflower over it. Scatter over the remaining breadcrumbs and cheese.
4. In the oven, bake the cauliflower cheese for twenty minutes until it bubbles.

Tip: Make enough for six servings, even if you need less as spare portions can be frozen before being baked.

PASTRY-LESS QUICHE

This is a very flexible recipe, since rather than the tomatoes, peppers, and mushrooms you can easily substitute all of the vegetables with any of your favorite vegetables, such as peas and dried mint or squash and sage. This dish can be eaten hot or cold as well, making it perfect for home dinner or for a packed lunch. Note that both mushrooms and tomatoes are high potassium foods, but ok when consumed in small amounts.

Serves 4

- One green pepper, diced
- One red pepper, diced
- One onion, chopped
- 75ml milk
- 50g (1¾oz) grated cheddar cheese or use a lower phosphate cheese such as feta
- Eight medium mushrooms, sliced
- 250g (9oz) fat free natural cottage cheese
- Two large or Three medium tomatoes, sliced
- Five eggs

Preparation method

1. Using a small amount of vegetable oil or spray oil to gently fry prepared vegetables (except tomatoes). You still want to make them a little crunchy, so don't overdo the veg.
2. Mix the 5 eggs, 250 g fat-free natural cottage cheese and the milk together-this is not a pretty combination, but stick with it.
3. In an oven-proof flan dish, spread the chopped vegetables out, then pour over the cottage cheese mix.
4. Place the sliced tomatoes on top and sprinkle the cheese on top.
5. Pop in the oven at 190 ° C (170 ° C fan)/375 ° F / Gas 5, for about thirty to forty-five minutes, or until the quiche is golden brown.

KIDNEY FRIENDLY PASTY

These pasties are great served hot from the oven, but in a packed lunch, they are equally tasty cold. In this recipe, we suggest par-boiling the swede and carrot, as this helps lower the potassium content of these vegetables.

Makes approximately six

- One medium carrot, peeled and chopped
- ½ small swede or ¼ large one, peeled and chopped
- 250g (8oz) of your chosen mince
- One medium onion, chopped finely
- Two teaspoons dried parsley
- 120ml low salt stock
- ½ teaspoon of English mustard
- 500g (17oz) ready-made short crust pastry
- Pepper
- One medium egg, lightly whisked

Preparation method

1. Pre-heat the oven to 180°C (160°C Fan)/350°F/ Gas 4.
2. The chopped swede and carrot are cooked on the hob for 5-10 minutes or until slightly soft. Drain and discard the water (this helps to reduce the potassium content of these vegetables). Let the vegetable to cool.
3. Add the parsley, minced beef, stock, onion, and English Mustard in a separate bowl.
4. To cut the minced beef into small strands, use a knife and mix the lot together with your hands to roughly spread the ingredients uniformly in the mixture. Season with pepper.
5. Add the cooled vegetables and blend gently with your mince mixture.
6. Roll the pastry out with a rolling pin to about 3mm thick. To leave a circle of pastry, press a saucer over the rolled pastry and cut through it. Then you can need to do three circles, reform the pastry and re-roll it. Place some of the filling on each circle.
7. Brush a little amount of the egg around the pastry's edges. To make a 'parcel' and crimp the edges together all the way round, put two edges of the pastry together.
8. Brush the egg on the sides of the pasties (to give the pasties a brown color during cooking).
9. Place the pasties in the pre-heated oven on a greased baking tray for fifty-five minutes.

LASAGNE

In general, lasagne includes two high potassium foods, milk and tomatoes, making it an avoidable dish for those who want to follow a low potassium diet to. We used soya milk in this recipe, which produces an almost tasty white sauce but is lower in potassium than cow's milk. You might also want some grated mozzarella cheese to top up your lasagne, which is a lower phosphate alternative to cheddar cheese.

Serves 3-4

- One tbsp of vegetable or olive oil
- 250g (9oz) of your chosen mince
- One onion, diced
- 750ml soya milk
- Two garlic cloves, crushed
- Three carrots, grated
- 75g (2½oz) butter or low fat spread
- 1 x 400g (14oz) tin of chopped tomatoes
- 75g (2½oz) plain flour
- One tsp English mustard
- One low salt stock cube (vegetable or beef)
- One tsp oregano or basil (optional)
- Pepper
- 100ml water
- 250g (9oz) lasagne sheets
- One large handful of grated mozzarella (optional)

Preparation method

1. Preheat the oven to 200°C (180°C Fan)/Gas /400°F6
2. Over a medium heat, heat a large frying pan and add the olive oil or the oil spray. Add your mince along with a good pinch of pepper once hot. Brown the mince for five to six minutes until it is colored all over and begins to crisp. Take the mince out of the pan and set it to one side.

3. Add the carrot and onion to the frying pan. Cook gently for ten minutes, or until everything is softened.

4. Meanwhile, over medium heat, melt the butter or spread it in a saucepan. When it has melted, add the flour and mustard and stir well to mix. Leave to cook for 2 minutes over medium heat, or until mixture makes a paste.

5. Pour the soya milk into the saucepan, whisking as you add to create a smooth white sauce. When you have applied a pinch of black pepper to all the soy milk, turn the heat down and let it simmer very gently for 7 minutes.

6. Add the garlic to the frying pan once the onions and carrots have softened and cook for 2 minutes. Return the meat (plus any juices) and add the tomatoes, stock and water back into the pan. Mix all together, cover with a lid and let the sauce simmer for ten minutes until slightly thickened.

7. Place a quarter of the tomato sauce into the bottom of a medium/small baking dish to assemble the lasagne. Cover with a lasagne sheet layer. Spoon the tomato sauce over another quarter and top it with a portion of the white sauce. Repeat this two more times, ending with the last layer of white sauce at the top.

8. Dish with the grated mozzarella

9. Put in the preheated oven and bake for thirty minutes or until the top is bubbling and golden brown.

HOMEMADE GRANOLA

Many shop bought granolas are unsuited if you are following phosphate and potassium restrictions due to the high content of dried fruit and nuts. To make your own alternative oat meal, here is an simple recipe that can be served with yogurt, stewed fruits, or milk. Here we have added dried cranberries as they are lower in potassium than other dried fruits; however, it will taste equally good without.

Makes up to ten servings

- Four tablespoons of vegetable oil or sunflower oil
- One lemon juice table spoon
- Two tablespoons of brown soft sugar
- Two tablespoons clear honey or golden syrup
- Dried cranberries (optional)

- 300g (10½oz) rolled oats

Preparation method

1. Preheat the oven to 140 ° C (120 ° C Fan)/275 ° F / Gas 1.
2. The oil, syrup/honey, lemon juice and sugar are melted in a large saucepan over a low heat. The intention is not to allow the mixture to bubble, only to allow the ingredients to melt and blend together. Then add the oats and stir thoroughly.
3. Spread the mixture in an even layer on a baking tray (depending on their size, you will need two baking trays. Bake in the oven until crisp for around 30-40 minutes. Check the granola every ten minutes and stir to ensure an even bake.
4. You can add a few handfuls of dried cranberries once cooked and cooled. The granola should be kept in an airtight container and utilized within one month.

TOAD IN THE HOLE

Treating yourself to some great quality sausages from the deli or butcher counter will help minimize the amount of additives often added to more processed foods. Adding low potassium flavorings such as mustard is a great way to spice up the sausages.

Serves 4

- ½ tsp English mustard powder
- 100g (3½oz) plain flour
- One egg
- Three thyme sprigs, leaves only (optional)
- 300ml milk
- Two tbsp of vegetable or olive oil
- Eight sausages

Preparation method:

1. Heat the oven to 220°C (200°C Fan)/Gas 7/425°F.
2. Tip the flour and whisk in the mustard powder in a large mixing bowl. In the center,

make a well, crack the egg, then pour a dribble of milk in. Stir with a wooden spoon until you have a smooth batter in the well, progressively adding some of the flour. Now add a little more milk and stir until you have mixed both the milk and flour together.

3. Now you should have a smooth, lump-free batter that is the consistency of double cream. Tip it into the jug in which you measured your milk, then stir in the thyme if using, for easier pouring later on.

4. To snip the ties between your sausages, use scissors, then drop them into a 20 x 30 cm roasting tin. Add 1 tablespoon of oil, toss in the sausages to coat the base of the tin thoroughly, then roast in the oven.

5. Remove the hot tray from the oven, then pour in the batter quickly. When it first reaches the hot fat, it should sizzle and bubble a little. Put it back in the oven, then bake for forty minutes until the batter is cooked through, well crisp. If you poke the tip of a knife into the batter in the center of the tray, It should be set, not runny or sticky.

PROVENCAL VEGETABLES WITH RICE
Nutritional values

Energy 357.5 kcal / Protein 10 g / P (phosphorus) 139.8 mg / K (potassium) 673.2 mg / Na (sodium) 18.4 mg

Ingredients

- pumpkin 250 g
- onion 50 g
- pepper 25 g
- zucchini 65 g
- tomatoes 125 g
- olive oil 5 ml
- rice 50 g
- pepper, Provencal herbs, garlic (or rosemary)

Method

Wash the vegetables, peel and remove the grains (tomatoes, peppers, pumpkins) and cut into cubes. In olive oil, fry the onion and garlic in olive oil. When slightly browned, add the other ingredients in this order: zucchini, peppers, Provencal herbs and pepper, pumpkin. Lightly fry with occasional stirring. Add the tomatoes, cover and cook on low heat for about an hour. Then turn the vegetables carefully and cook (fry) for the last 10 minutes. Sprinkle with chopped parsley and serve with rice.

TUNA PASTA BAKE

This is a perfect recipe for a brisk supper and you may have all the ingredients in the fridge/cupboard already.

Serves 4

- 25g (1oz) olive oil spread or unsalted butter
- 25g (1oz) plain flour
- ½ tsp mustard or mustard powder
- 200g (7oz) cream cheese
- 400ml milk
- Pepper
- Handful of each; sweet corn and pea
- 130g (4½oz) canned tuna, drained and flaked
- ½ onion, peeled, finely chopped
- 60-80g (2-3oz) dried breadcrumbs (shop brought or homemade)
- 160g (5½oz) pasta (such as penne, fusilli, or macaroni), cooked according to packet instructions, drained

Preparation method:

1. Preheat oven to 200°C (180°C Fan)/Gas 6/400°F.
2. Heat the spread or butter in a frying pan over a medium heat. To make a smooth paste, add the flour when the butter is foaming. Continue to cook, stirring vigorously, then

pour in 125ml/4½fl oz of milk for another three - four minutes. Whisk the flour and milk mixture to a smooth paste.

3. Add another 125ml/4½fl oz of milk while the mixture is bubbling and whisk until it bubbles and is absorbed into the mixture.

4. Repeat this with the remaining 250ml/9fl oz of milk. Keep whisking and boil until smooth and thick enough for the back of a spoon to cover the sauce. Stir in the cream cheese and remove the pan from the heat. Season with mustard and pepper.

5. Add the tuna, peas, onion, cooked pasta and sweet corn to the cheese sauce and stir until well mixed.

6. In an ovenproof dish, pour the mixture into it. Sprinkle the breadcrumbs over it. Bake for thirty minutes in the oven, or until the breadcrumbs are golden brown and crisp and the sauce bubbling.

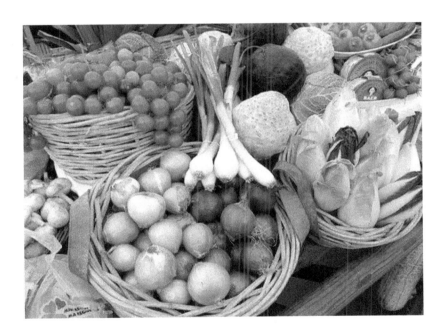

CHAPTER 7: VEGAN DISHES

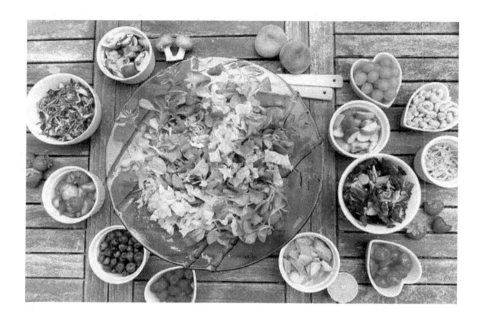

CARROT AND CORIANDER SOUP

Carrots are a delicious low potassium vegetable, plus the use of a low salt stock ensures that it is kidney friendly. Remember that soup is fluid, so count it if you are on a fluid restriction.

Serves four

- 450g (1lb) carrots, sliced
- One tbsp of vegetable or olive oil
- One tsp ground coriander
- One onion, sliced
- 1.2 litres/2 pints vegetable stock such as low salt Bouillon
- Large bunch fresh parsley or fresh coriander, roughly chopped (optional)
- One bay leaf

- Freshly ground black pepper

Preparation method

1. In a large pan, heat the oil and add the onions and carrots. Cook for 3-4 minutes before softening begins.
2. Stir in the ground coriander and season properly. One minute to cook.
3. Add the vegetable stock and bay leaf and bring to the boil. Simmer until the vegetables are tender.
4. Remove the bay leaf and use a hand blender or a blender to whizz the soup until smooth. In a clean pan, reheat. Stir in the fresh parsley or coriander and serve with some crusty bread.

HEALTHY CHIPS

These chips are lower in potassium because they are parboiled, so good if you adopt a low potassium diet. They are healthier if you use less oil, so the spray oil is perfect if you want to lose weight.

Serves 4

- A small amount of vegetable, spray oil or olive oil
- 908g (2lb) medium sized Maris Piper potatoes

Preparation method

1. Preheat oven to 240°C (220°C Fan)/Gas 9/475°F. Peel the potatoes with a potato peeler, then remove any blemishes. Slice into approx ½in/1cm thick rectangular chips.
2. Bring a big saucepan of salted water to a boil. Add your chips and cook for four minutes. Drain and leave it aside for ten minutes to dry.
3. Put the chips back to the dry saucepan, cover it with a lid and shake the edges of the chips to rough the edges. This roughness is vital to the chips' texture.
4. Lightly grease the olive oil or spray oil on the metal baking tray. Bake in the oven for twenty minutes, turning periodically, until golden brown on all sides. Move the chips

to the tray, spray lightly with oil spray or cover lightly with olive oil. Drain on absorbent kitchen paper and serve.

PIZZA BIANCA

Nutritional values per serving

Energy 101 kcal, Protein 2 g, BE 1, Fat 4 g, Carbohydrates 14 g, Potassium 36 mg, Phosphorus 21 mg

Ingredients for 8 pieces:

- For the dough 150 g Wheat flour type 405
- 1 teaspoon (5g) sugar
- 10 g yeast
- 100 ml lukewarm water
- 1 tbsp (10g) olive oil
- ½ tsp salt

For covering

- 2 tbsp (20g) olive oil
- 1 teaspoon (4g) oregano or pizza seasoning

Method

Dissolve the yeast with the sugar in the water, then add to the flour with oil and salt and knead into a smooth dough.

Put the dough in a bowl and dust with flour. Cover the bowl with foil, let the dough rise in a warm place until the volume has doubled.

Knead the risen dough vigorously again. Form 8 small balls from the mass. Line an oven tray with baking paper, roll out each ball into a small round pizza. Let everything go a second time.

Mix the oil with the herbs and brush the pizza with it. Bake in the preheated oven at 200

° C for 5 to 10 minutes.

TZATZIKI
Nutritional values per serving

Energy 162 kcal, Protein 11 g, Potassium 193 mg, Phosphorus 154 mg

Ingredients for 6 servings

- 500 g Quark
- 1 cucumber
- 4th Garlic cloves
- salt
- 2 tbsp vinegar
- 3 tbsp Sunflower oil

Method

Grate the cucumber, season with salt and let it steep. Squeeze out the juice and discard.

Mix the quark with salt, vinegar and oil, add the squeezed garlic and squeezed cucumber, season to taste.

OBATZDA
Nutritional values per serving

Energy 230 kcal, Protein 12 g, Potassium 120 mg, Phosphorus 140 mg

Ingredients for 6 servings:

- 200 g well matured Camembert 40% fat i. Tr.
- 3 tbsp Quark
- 1 finely chopped shallot
- 40 g soft butter

- Pepper
- 1 Mocha spoon sweet paprika
- 2 red radishes finely diced
- 1 tbsp Spring onion finely diced
- 1 tbsp Chive rolls

Method

Mash the camembert and butter well in a bowl until an almost homogeneous mass is formed.

Then add the other ingredients and season to taste.

APPLE SORBET
Nutritional values

Energy 75.3 kcal / Protein 0.5 g / P (phosphorus) 15 mg / K (potassium) 175 mg / Na (sodium) 8 mg

Ingredients

- apples 125 g
- sugar 5 g (1 teaspoon)
- lemon juice 5 ml (1 teaspoon)
- water 50 ml

Method

Let it boil water with sugar. Peel and grate the apples or cut them finely. Add them to the water together with the lemon juice, cook for 2-3 minutes and mix. The resulting mixture is passed through a sieve, allowed to cool and put in the freezer. We mix just before serving, when we can decorate to taste. Tip: Can be made with any other fruit.

APPLESAUCE
Nutritional values

Energy 73 kcal / Protein 0.6 g / P (phosphorus) 18 mg / K (potassium) 210 mg / Na (sodium) 9 mg

Ingredients

- sour apple 1 pc
- sugar 2 g
- star anise

Method

Cut the cleaned apple into cubes, cover with water, add star anise, sugar and stew. Allow to cool, mix and serve.

BAKED APPLES
Nutritional values

Energy 411.5 kcal / Protein 2.8 g / P (phosphorus) 65.6 mg / K (potassium) 256.1 mg / Na (sodium) 9.9 mg

Ingredients

- low-protein biscuits 10 g
- low-protein waffles 30 g
- apple 125 g
- peeled almonds 10 g
- sugar 15 g
- fat 10 g

Method

Grate almonds, mix low-protein biscuits with sugar and melted fat. Wash the apple and cut it around the entire perimeter, removing the core. Put the filling in the hole after the core. Bake in a greased dish. Sprinkle the hot apple with sugar and serve on a waffle. We can decorate the apple with whipped cream. Instead of sugar, we can add homemade jam to the filling, grate the lemon peel and season with cinnamon.

CHARD SALAD
Nutritional values

Energy 37.3 kcal / Protein 1.2 g / P (phosphorus) 24.5 mg / K (potassium) 210 mg / Na (sodium) 46.4 mg

Ingredients

- chard 50 g
- onion 10 g
- sugar 5 g
- vinegar
- chive

Method

Remove the leaves of the chard leaves, peel them off and cut them into smaller pieces, which we boil in salted water. Drain and allow to cool in a bowl. Pour the marinade prepared from vinegar, salt, oil, sugar and water over the cold chard. Garnish with chopped chives.

FENNEL SALAD
Nutritional values

Energy 34.2 kcal / Protein 1.3 g / P (phosphorus) 2 mg / K (potassium) 9.6 mg / Na (sodium) 393.5 mgIngredients

Ingredients

- fennel 50 g
- onion 5 g
- sugar 5 g
- lemon juice
- salt

Method

Cut the cleaned petals of fennel into shorter pieces (or grate) and pour over the dressing, which we prepare from water, sugar, lemon juice and salt.

CELERY SALAD
Nutritional values

Energy 73.9 kcal / Protein 1.1 g / P (phosphorus) 49.4 mg / K (potassium) 268.7 mg / Na (sodium) 71 mg

Ingredients

- celery 70 g
- onion 15 g
- sugar 2 g
- oil 5 g
- bay leaf, vinegar

Method

Peel a celery and an onion and cut into slices. We then cook them with spices. After cooking, drain and acidify with vinegar and sweeten. Add oil. Serve in a salad bowl.

CHICORY PUCK SALAD
Nutritional values

Energy 62.3 kcal / Protein 1.4 g / P (phosphorus) 29.3 mg / K (potassium) 313.9 mg / Na (sodium) 96 mg

Ingredients

- chicory buds 65 g
- apple 40 g
- orange 25 g
- lemon juice
- sugar 5 g
- Salt

Method

We clean the chicory buds, cut them into fine strips and let them rest. Drain the infused bitter juice. Peel an apple and cut it into cubes. Peel an orange and peel the flesh, which we cut into small pieces. We mix chicory buds with cubes of apples and oranges. Drizzle the salad with lemon juice, lightly salt, season with sugar and mix well.

JAMAICA SALAD
Nutritional values

Energy 60.8 kcal / Protein 1.3 g / P (phosphorus) 32.6 mg / K (potassium) 261 mg / Na (sodium) 90 mg

Ingredients

- lettuce 25 g
- orange 25 g
- pineapple 25 g

- kiwi 25 g
- orange juice (100%) 50 ml
- salt

Method

Wash the lettuce well and cut it into smaller pieces. Remove the skin, kiwi and pineapple from the skins and inedible parts and cut into small cubes. Mix together and pour over slightly salted orange juice.

SPAGHETTI WITH ZUCCHINI
Nutritional values

Energy 279.7 kcal / Protein 5.7 g / P (phosphorus) 46 mg / K (potassium) 167.3 mg / Na (sodium) 3.2 mg

Ingredients

- low-protein spaghetti 50 g
- green zucchini 25 g
- tomato salsa (crushed tomatoes with herbs) 30 ml
- garlic 1 g
- olive oil 10 ml
- sage

Method

Cut the zucchini into slices, cut the garlic into small cubes or squeeze. Fry everything in oil with sage. Add salsa and cooked pasta to bite. Let it warm up for a few minutes and sprinkle with fresh chopped parsley before serving.

FRUIT HOT CUP
Nutritional values

Energy 229.3 kcal / Protein 1.1 g / P (phosphorus) 36.5 mg / K (potassium) 214.9 mg / Na (sodium) 12.6 mg

Ingredients

- apple (smaller) 1 pc
- raspberries 50 g
- low-protein biscuits 40 g
- starch 5 g
- vanilla sugar
- cinnamon

Method

Peel an apple, cut into thin slices, drizzle with water. We stew apples even with spices until soft. Mix the starch in a little water and pour the stewed apples and cook lightly. This is how we prepare raspberries. We alternately place a porridge of apples and raspberries and broken sponge cakes in the cup.

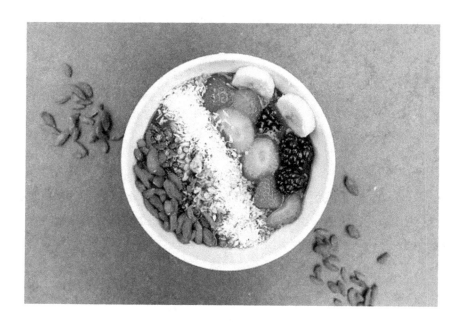

CHEESE SPREAD
Nutritional values

Energy 132 kcal / Protein 4.8 g / P (phosphorus) 76 mg / K (potassium) 31 mg / Na (sodium) 141 mg

Ingredients

- eidam 30% 15 g
- vegetable fat 12 g
- garlic, salt, curry, chives to taste

Method

Rub butter in a bowl, add grated cheese and garlic. Lightly salt, add curry spice and chopped chives. Serve on toast.

TUNA SPREAD
Nutritional values

Energy 173 kcal / Protein 16 g / P (phosphorus) 120 mg / K (potassium) 170 mg / Na (sodium) 191 mg

Ingredients

- tuna (canned in its own juice) 50 g
- Lučiny 50 g
- onion 30 g
- lemon juice
- chive

Method

Grind the tuna with Lucina to the foam and add to the finely chopped onion. Season with lemon juice and garnish with chives. Serve with bread.

ITALIAN BRUSCHETTA (TOAST)
Nutritional values

Energy 124.8 kcal / Protein 3.4 g / P (phosphorus) 56 mg / K (potassium) 331.7 mg / Na (sodium) 134.2 mg

Ingredients

- ripe tomatoes 100 g
- white bread 25 g
- olive oil 5 ml
- garlic 5 g
- white pepper ¼ g (pinch)

Method

Bake the bread, sprinkle with garlic and drizzle with olive oil. Put ripe tomatoes, diced and pepper.

AVOCADO SPREAD
Nutritional values

Energy 240 kcal / Protein 5 g / P (phosphorus) 32 mg / K (potassium) 309 mg / Na (sodium) 3 mg

Ingredients

- avocado 50 g
- Lučina 50g
- red onion small
- garlic clove

- salt

Method

Wash the avocado. We halve it and stone it. We dig out the contents with a spoon. We mix it with a fork together with Lučina, finely chopped onion and crushed garlic. Lightly salt.

MEXICAN POTATO SALAD
Nutritional values

Energy 212.9 kcal / Protein 2.6 g / P (phosphorus) 68.5 mg / K (potassium) 628.3 mg / Na (sodium) 18.6 mg

Ingredients

- potatoes 75 g
- tomatoes 100 g
- onion 5 g
- garlic 0.2 g
- parsley leaf 0.2 g
- rapeseed oil 15 ml

Method

Peeled potatoes cut into slices and cook until soft, drain and put in a serving bowl. Drizzle them immediately with vinegar and allow to cool. Once the potatoes are cold, add the chopped (very ripe) tomatoes, chopped onion, garlic and rapeseed oil and mix gently to combine. Season and sprinkle with chopped parsley. Serve at room temperature.

ITALIAN NOODLES WITH CHEESE
Nutritional values

Energy 434.8 kcal / Protein 8.4 g / P (phosphorus) 224.2 mg / K (potassium) 116.6 mg / Na (sodium) 202.6 mg

Ingredients

- low-protein noodles 80 g
- onion 20 g
- olive oil 15 g + 5 g
- tomato puree 20 g
- parmesan 20 g
- salt, pepper, garlic, parsley

Method

Fry the onion and add the puree, crushed garlic and parsley. Pour boiled noodles into the heated base and mix. Serve in a deep plate and sprinkle with grated cheese and drizzle with olive oil.

SALMON ROLLS
Nutritional values

Energy 293.2 kcal / Protein 22.1 g / P (phosphorus) 281 mg / K (potassium) 730 mg / Na (sodium) 76 mg

Ingredients

- 2 thin slices of salmon (one around 50 g) 100 g
- frozen spinach 100 g
- Solamyl (+ water) 5 g
- oil 10 g
- salt pepper

Method

Thaw the spinach and squeeze the water. Then thicken with solamyl and season with pepper and salt. Brush the slice of salmon with spinach and wrap it in a roll. Close the roll with a needle and fry in warm oil and bake until soft. (solamyl is also potato powder)

LETTUCE
Nutritional values

Energy 49.2 kcal / Protein 0.8 g / P (phosphorus) 20.2 mg / K (potassium) 148.5 mg / Na (sodium) 10 mg

Ingredients

- lettuce 1/4 pc
- water
- vinegar
- sugar
- oil

Method

Wash the lettuce and cut it into smaller pieces. Prepare the dressing in a bowl - let the sugar dissolve in the water and then add the vinegar and oil. Finally, mix the salad with the dressing and we're done.

APRICOT ACID
Nutritional values

Energy 139.1 kcal / Protein 0.7 g / P (phosphorus) 21 mg / K (potassium) 250 mg / Na (sodium) 3 mg

Ingredients

- apricot compote without juice 150 g
- solamyl 5 g

Method

Remove the apricots from the compote, mix. Boil the mixed apricots, add solamyl mixed in a small amount of cold water and cook.

FRIED POTATOES
Nutritional values

Energy 300.6 kcal / Protein 5 g / P (phosphorus) 130 mg / K (potassium) 1 130 mg / Na (sodium) 40 mg

Ingredients

- potatoes 250 g
- water
- oil 10 g
- caraway seeds
- salt pinch

Method

Wash the potatoes and cook softly with the peel. After cooling, peel them and cut them into wheels. Then fry the potatoes in a hot pan with a little oil.

ROASTED CARROTS
Nutritional values

Energy 89.1 kcal / Protein 1.1 g / P (phosphorus) 42 mg / K (potassium) 289.5 mg / Na (sodium) 87.8 mg

Ingredients

- carrot 100 g
- margarine 10 g

- onion 5 g
- parsley leaf 1 g

Method

Peel a carrot and clean the onion. We cut both. Heat the margarine in a pan and fry the onion on it first, then add the carrots and fry for about 10 minutes. Sprinkle with chopped parsley and serve either as a side dish or a separate meal.

STEAMED RICE WITH STERILIZED PEAS
Nutritional values

Energy 317.3 kcal / Protein 6.3 g / P (phosphorus) 104.7 mg / K (potassium) 116.2 mg / Na (sodium) 76.7 mg

Ingredients

- rice 80 g
- sterilized peas 15 g
- onion 5 g
- water 120 ml
- oil 3 g

Method

Rinse the rice. Pour water over it and cook it until soft together with the onion and salt. Drain the cooked rice and mix with the oil and peas.

POTATO SOUP
Nutritional values

Energy 134.8 kcal / Protein 1.6 g / P (phosphorus) 31.5 mg / K (potassium) 166.7 mg / Na (sodium) 9.1 mg

Ingredients

- potatoes 30 g
- frozen vegetables 50 g
- fresh mushrooms 10 g
- oil 10 g
- marjoram, pepper, chives, crushed cumin, garlic, a pinch of salt

Method

Peel the potatoes and cut into small cubes. Fry frozen vegetables and potatoes in oil. Pour water over the roasted mixture, add mushrooms cut into smaller pieces, spices and crushed garlic. We cook everything until soft. Finally, add the chopped chives. We can soften the soup with butter, which we add to the finished soup.

CHAPTER 8: OTHER DISHES

PORK AFTER GARDENING
Nutritional values

Energy 386.5 kcal / Protein 17.3 g / P (phosphorus) 189 mg / K (potassium) 355.5 mg / Na (sodium) 71.5 mg

Ingredients

- lean pork 85 g
- vegetable mixture 100 g
- onion 10 g
- butter 5 g
- oil 10 g
- potato starch (+ water) 5 g
- salt, pepper, cumin, parsley

Method

Fry the onion in oil, add the meat cut into strips. Pour water over the meat and simmer until semi-soft. Add vegetables cut into circles, spices and stew together. Before finishing, thicken with a mixture of potato starch and water. Soften the dish with fresh butter and parsley.

POTATO SALAD WITH APPLES
Nutritional values

Energy 502 kcal / Protein 7 g / P (phosphorus) 181 mg / K (potassium) 777 mg / Na (sodium) 0 mg

Ingredients

- potatoes 200 g
- eggs ½
- apple 1
- onions 1
- Dijon mustard ce spoon
- mayonnaise 50 g
- lemon, salt, pepper

Method

Peel the boiled potatoes and cut into larger cubes, put in a bowl. (Patients who monitor their potassium levels first peel the potatoes, cut them into cubes and leave them soaked in water for at least 2 hours, then cook in new water). Add sliced cucumbers and eggs to the potatoes. Grate the onion and the apple on a coarse grater. Mix everything with mayonnaise, mustard, lemon pepper. juice and served with roast.

ROAST PORK WITH CHANTERELLES
Nutritional values

Energy 354 kcal / Protein 15 g / P (phosphorus) 203 mg / K (potassium) 561 mg / Na (sodium) 0 mg

Ingredients

- neck 70 g

- multicolored pepper
- foxes 50 g
- shallots 1
- oil 1 tbsp
- butter 1 tbsp
- parsley ¼ bundle

Method

Rub salt and pepper into the meat. Leave to rest for an hour and then fry the meat on all sides in oil. Roast the meat at 180 ° C for about 45 minutes to keep it pink and juicy in the middle. If necessary, cover it with a little water during baking and pour over the baked juice. Remove the soft roast from the baking and keep warm until you finish the juice. Meanwhile, fry in half a tablespoon of fox butter along with a white portion of onions. Strain the juice, stir in the cold leftover butter and add the roasted chanterelles with onions. Cut the meat into slices and serve with juice.

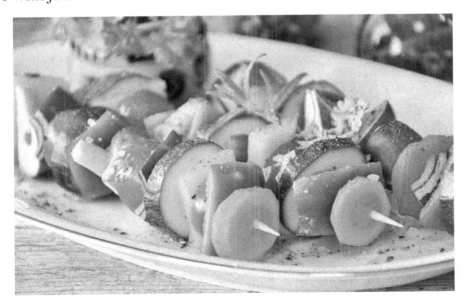

CHICKEN ON LEMON AND HONEY
Nutritional values

Energy 228 kcal / Protein 18 g / P (phosphorus) 176 mg / K (potassium) 252 mg / Na (sodium) 121 mg

Ingredients

- 2 chicken breasts - size 80 g (per serving)
- 1 tablespoon honey, finely grated rind
- and the juice of one smaller lemon
- 1 tablespoon olive oil, salt, pepper
- crispy cabbage salad

Method

Preheat the oven to 190 ° C. Spread the washed breast in a baking dish, baking dish. Beat the juice, peel, pepper, oil, salt and pour over the meat. Turn the chicken in the marinade several times to wrap it thoroughly. Tip - you can have the meat marinated for a few hours - it depends on your time Bake the chicken breasts for about 20 minutes, then turn them over and bake for another 20 minutes and occasionally spread the juice. After roasting, let the meat cool down for a very short time and cut the breast into thin slices, which you add to the meat juice. Serve on torn salad leaves and choose orange rice as a side dish.

CABBAGE ROLLS WITH MINCED MEAT
Nutritional values

Energy 339 kcal / Protein 15 g / P (phosphorus) 163 mg / K (potassium) 574 mg / Na (sodium) 53 mg

Ingredients

- 1 piece of cabbage
- minced meat - mixed 250 g
- 1 kitchen onion
- 1 clove of garlic
- 5 pcs cherry tomatoes
- 1 teaspoon - ground cumin, sl. peppers, thyme, oregano
- oil 50 g

- vegetable broth - for drizzling

Method

Wash the cabbage, dry it, break off the upper larger leaves, cut a hard broom out of them and immerse them in boiling water for 2 minutes. Then let them cool. In a casserole, fry in 2 tablespoons of oil and add the minced meat and the rest of the grated cabbage, sliced tomatoes. Season the mixture with spices and salt and simmer briefly while stirring constantly. Fill the cabbage leaves with the finished mixture, twist them tightly and transport them with food string. Wipe the baking tray with the rest of the oil and spread out the cabbage rolls and add a few thin slices of butter to soften. Bake under the lid for about 15 minutes at a temperature of 180 ° C, then uncover the rolls and bake briefly until they are slightly golden in color. The ideal side dish is boiled or baked potatoes or low-protein bread. Tip - Instead of meat it is possible to use Balkan cheese or bacon, rice. It is possible to add sterilized peeled tomatoes to the baking dish and stew them together with rolls.

CHICKEN SOUP WITH RICE NOODLES
Nutritional values

Energy 124 kcal / Protein 8 g / P (phosphorus) 157 mg / K (potassium) 249 mg / Na (sodium) 67 mg

Ingredients

- root vegetables (ideally frozen at high levels of potassium) 40 g
- chicken meat, cut into cubes 30 g
- sunflower oil 3 g
- onion 5 g
- Clove of garlic
- water (or vegetable broth) 400 ml
- rice noodles 15 g
- Parsley and celery leaves, whole pepper, salt

Method

Fry the cleaned vegetables in oil, pour water (broth) and add diced meat, tops and spices. Cook until the meat softens. Add cooked rice noodles to the finished soup and garnish with parsley. Rice noodles - cook in salted boiling water until soft, then drain.

FRIED CHICKEN SCHNITZEL
Nutritional values

Energy 327 kcal / Protein 13 g / P (phosphorus) 126 mg / K (potassium) 159 mg / Na (sodium) 56 mg

Ingredients

- chicken breast 45 g
- eggs 1
- NB flour 10 g
- NB crumbs 10 g
- vegetable oil for frying 20 ml
- salt pepper

Method

Tap the meat, salt and pepper. We gradually wrap it in flour, then in an egg and finally in breadcrumbs. After wrapping, put the meat in hot oil and wait for it to roast until golden on both sides. Finally, we can drizzle with lemon.

CHICKEN ON ROSEMARY
Nutritional values

Energy 287 kcal / Protein 21.6 g / P (phosphorus) 180.7 mg / K (potassium) 355.7 mg / Na (sodium) 143 mg

Ingredients

- slice of chicken 70 g
- onion 50 g
- oil 20 g
- lemon juice
- rosemary spoon
- salt pinch
- pepper, lemon peel

Method

Tap a slice of chicken lightly, season with (rosemary, salt, pepper and lemon zest) and fry vigorously on both sides. Add the chopped onion to the roasted meat and bake until soft. Finally, taste with lemon juice.

BEEF IN CARROTS
Nutritional values

Energy 269.8 kcal / Protein 12.6 g / P (phosphorus) 131.5 mg / K (potassium) 456 mg / Na (sodium) 112.9 mg

Ingredients

- lean beef 50 g
- carrot 100 g
- plain flour 15 g
- quality vegetable oil 15 g

Method

Cut the cleaned meat into cubes, fry in oil. Add cleaned and chopped carrots, cover with water and simmer gently. Dust with flour and cook properly.

PORK AFTER GARDENING
Nutritional values

Energy 386.5 kcal / Protein 17.3 g / P (phosphorus) 189 mg / K (potassium) 355.5 mg / Na (sodium) 71.5 mg

Ingredients

- lean pork 85 g
- vegetable mixture 100 g
- onion 10 g
- butter 5 g
- oil 10 g
- potato starch (+ water) 5 g
- salt, pepper, cumin, parsley

Method

Fry the onion in oil, add the meat cut into strips. Pour water over the meat and simmer until semi-soft. Add vegetables cut into circles, spices and stew together. Before finishing, thicken with a mixture of potato starch and water. Soften the dish with fresh butter and parsley.

ROAST PORK WITH CHANTERELLES
Nutritional values

Energy 354 kcal / Protein 15 g / P (phosphorus) 203 mg / K (potassium) 561 mg / Na (sodium) 0 mg

Ingredients

- neck 70 g
- multicolored pepper

- foxes 50 g
- shallots 1
- oil 1 tbsp
- butter 1 tbsp
- parsley ¼ bundle

Method

Rub salt and pepper into the meat. Leave to rest for an hour and then fry the meat on all sides in oil. Roast the meat at 180 ° C for about 45 minutes to keep it pink and juicy in the middle. If necessary, cover it with a little water during baking and pour over the baked juice. Remove the soft roast from the baking and keep warm until you finish the juice. Meanwhile, fry in half a tablespoon of fox butter along with a white portion of onions. Strain the juice, stir in the cold leftover butter and add the roasted chanterelles with onions. Cut the meat into slices and serve with juice.

PORK ON PEPPER
Nutritional values

Energy 406.6 kcal / Protein 12.7 g / P (phosphorus) 11.4 mg / K (potassium) 30.8 mg / Na (sodium) 43.5 mg

Ingredients

- pork medium fat 80 g
- onion 15 g
- oil 15 g
- potato starch 7 g
- water or vegetable broth
- ground pepper 2 balls
- salt

Method

Fry the onion in oil and fry until pink. Add the meat and fry on both sides. Drizzle the meat with water or vegetable broth, add pepper and simmer until soft. Concentrate the juice with potato starch. Cook and serve.

PORK IN CHINESE
Nutritional values

Energy 295 kcal / Protein 10.2 g / P (phosphorus) 106 mg / K (potassium) 197.5 mg / Na (sodium) 40.2 mg

Ingredients

- pork lean meat 50 g
- frozen vegetables chinese mixture 100 g
- quality vegetable oil 15 g
- solamyl 5 g(potato powder)

Method

We clean the meat, cut it into strips, wrap it in solamyl. Fry the meat in a hot pan. Then add vegetables, a small amount of water and stew. Lightly salt.

OYSTER MUSHROOM SOUP
Nutritional values

Energy 223.9 kcal / Protein 2.9 g / P (phosphorus) 54.9 mg / K (potassium) 244.4 mg / Na (sodium) 205.7 mg

Ingredients

- oyster mushrooms 60 g

- onion 30 g
- meat broth 100 ml
- starch 10 g
- oil 15 ml
- sweet pepper 1 g
- salt 0.5 g
- pepper 0.5 g

Method

Stew the chopped onion for about 5 minutes in 2 tablespoons of water. Add chopped mushrooms and continue for 5 min. Add 100 ml of broth and spices, cover with a lid and cook for another 15 minutes at low temperature. While the mushrooms are suffocating, heat the oil in a pot and mix the starch well into it with a whisk. Pour water and whisk the mixture to a thick and creamy consistency. Let it simmer for about 10 minutes at low temperatures and with frequent stirring. Add the finished mixture to the mushrooms and simmer for another 10 minutes. If necessary, add water and spices.

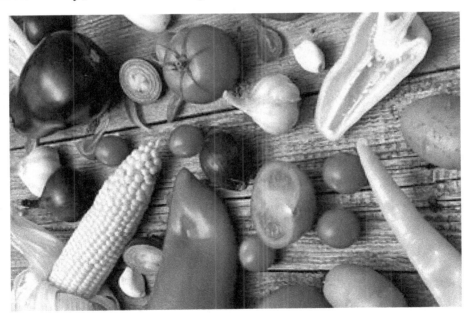

CHAPTER 9: ADOPTING A NEW LIFESTYLE TO REDUCE YOUR KIDNEY PROBLEMS

Kidney diseases are silent killers that can affect the quality of life to a large extent. There are many ways that the risk of developing kidney disease can be reduced.

Keep fit, Be active

This will help maintain the optimum weight of your body, decrease your blood pressure, and reduce your risk of Chronic Kidney Disease.

The idea of "On the move for kidney health" is a joint march around the world involving the public, celebrities and practitioners walking, running and cycling around a public field. Why not join them!

Eat a healthy diet

This will help maintain an optimum weight for the body, minimize blood pressure, heart disease, prevent diabetes, and other Chronic Kidney Disease-related conditions.

Reduce your salt consumption. 5-6 grams of salt per day is the optimal sodium intake. This includes the salt already in your foods. Try to minimize the amount of processed and restaurant food and do not add salt to food in order to reduce the salt intake. Controlling your salt consumption would be easier if you cook the food yourself with fresh ingredients.

Check and control your blood sugar

About half of people with diabetes are unaware that they have diabetes. As part of your general body checkup, you therefore need to check your blood sugar level. For those who are approaching middle age or older, this is particularly important. Around half of people with diabetes experience kidney damage, but if the diabetes is well managed, this can be prevented / limited. Check your kidney function regularly with urine and blood tests.

Check and control your blood pressure

About half of people with high blood pressure are unaware that they have high blood pressure. As part of your general body checkup, you therefore need to check your blood pressure. For those who are reaching middle age or older, this is particularly important. Your kidneys can be impaired by high blood pressure. This is particularly probable in conjunction with other causes, such as diabetes , cardio-vascular diseases and high cholesterol. With good blood pressure control, the risk can be decreased.

The level of normal adult blood pressure is 120/80. Hypertension is diagnosed if the systolic blood pressure readings on both days reach ~140 mmHg and/or the diastolic blood pressure readings on both days reach ~90 mmHg (WHO) when measured on two different days.

If your blood pressure is persistently above the average range (especially if you are a young person), you should contact your doctor to address the risks, the need for lifestyle change and medication treatment.

The recommendations for high blood pressure (2017) were updated by the American Heart Association and the American College of Cardiology and indicated that high blood pressure should be treated sooner with lifestyle modifications and treatment at 130/80 mm Hg instead of 140/90 mm Hg. This suggestion, however, has not been accepted by all health organizations around the world. It's best to see a doctor.

Take appropriate fluid intake

For any individual, the right amount of fluid intake depends on several variables, including health conditions, pregnancy, breastfeeding, exercise, and climate.

In a comfortable climate, this typically means 8 cups, around 2 liters (quarts) per day for a healthy person.

This needs to be changed when the climate condition is severe. If you have kidney disease or liver or heart disease, you may need to alter your fluid intake. Consult your doctor about the fluid intake that is appropriate for your condition.

Don't smoke

Smoking slows down the flow of blood to the kidneys. It may decrease their ability to function normally as less blood enters the kidneys. Smoking also raises the risk of kidney cancer by about 50%.

Do not take over-the-counter pain-killer/anti-inflammatory tablets regularly.

Common drugs such as non-steroidal anti-inflammatory (NSAIDS)/ pain killers (for instance, drugs such as ibuprofen) can damage the kidneys if taken frequently.

Taking only a couple of doses will damage your kidneys if you have kidney disease or reduced kidney function. Consult your doctor or pharmacist if in doubt.

Get your kidney function checked, If you have one or more of the 'high risk' factors.

- you have hypertension
- you have diabetes
- you have a family history of kidney disease
- you are obese

CHAPTER 10: MANAGING RENAL DIET WHEN YOU ARE DIABETIC

————— ✌︎ —————

One of the most effective therapies in the managing kidney disease and diabetes is diet. You will need to work with a dietitian to develop an eating plan that's right for you if you have been diagnosed with kidney disease as a result of diabetes. This strategy will help control the levels of blood glucose and reduce the amount of waste and fluid processed by the kidneys.

Which nutrients do I need to regulate?

Your dietician will provide you with dietary instructions that tell you how much protein, fat , and carbohydrates you will consume, and how much potassium, sodium, and phosphorus you can consume each day. Since these minerals need to be lower in your diet, you can restrict or eliminate those foods when planning your meals.

Portion control is also important. Speak with your dietitian about tips for measuring a serving size accurately. What can be measured on a regular diet as one serving may count as three servings on the kidney diet.

In order to maintain your blood glucose at an even level, the doctor and dietitian will also recommend that you eat meals and snacks of the same size and carbohydrate/calorie content at certain times of the day. It is vital that blood glucose levels are always tested and the results are shared with your doctor.

What can I eat?

An example of food choices that are commonly recommended on a standard renal diabetic diet is given below. This list is focused on the inclusion of foods containing sodium, phosphorus, potassium, and high sugar content. Ask your dietitian if you can have any of the listed foods and ensure you know what the recommended serving size should be.

Carbohydrate Foods

Milk and nondairy

RECOMMENDED	AVOID
Non-dairy creamer, plain yogurt, skim or fat-free milk, sugar-free pudding, sugar-free ice cream, sugar-free yogurt, sugar-free nondairy frozen desserts* *Portions of dairy products are often limited to four ounces due to high potassium, phosphorus or protein content	Buttermilk, sweetened yogurt, chocolate milk, sugar sweetened, sugar sweetened ice cream, pudding, sugar sweetened nondairy frozen desserts

Breads and starches

RECOMMENDED	AVOID
Sourdough, whole grain bread and whole wheat, unsweetened, white, wheat, rye, cream of wheat, grits, malt-o-meal, rice, bagel (small), refined dry cereals, noodles, white or whole wheat pasta, cornbread (made from scratch), flour tortilla, hamburger bun, unsalted crackers	Frosted or sugar-coated cereals, bran bread, gingerbread, pancake mix, cornbread mix, instant cereals, bran or granola, biscuits, salted snacks including: potato chips, corn chips and crackers Whole wheat cereals like oatmeal, wheat flakes and raisin bran, and whole grain hot cereals contain more potassium and phosphorus than refined products.

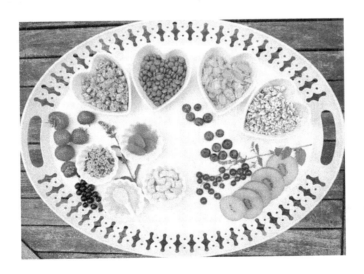

Fruits and juices

RECOMMENDED	AVOID
Applesauce, apricot halves, apples, apple juice, berries including: cranberries, blackberries and blueberries, strawberries, raspberries, low sugar cranberry juice, grapes, grape juice, kumquats, cherries, fruit cocktail, grapefruit, plums, tangerine, watermelon, mandarin oranges, pears, pineapple, fruit canned in unsweetened juice	Bananas, cantaloupe, avocados, dried fruits including: raisins, dates, and prunes, kumquats, star fruit, fresh pears, honeydew melon, kiwis, mangos, oranges and orange juice, papaya, nectarines, pomegranate, fruit canned in syrup

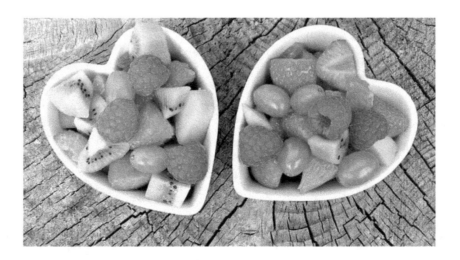

Starchy vegetables

RECOMMENDED	AVOID
Mixed vegetables with corn and peas (eat these less often because they are high in phosphorus), corn, peas, potatoes (soaked to reduce potassium)	Yams, baked beans, baked potatoes, sweet potatoes, dried beans (kidneys, pinto or soy, lima , lentil), succotash, winter squash, pumpkin

Non-starchy vegetables

RECOMMENDED	AVOID
Brussels sprouts, carrots, asparagus, beets, broccoli, cabbage, cauliflower, celery, cucumber, green beans, iceberg lettuce, eggplant, frozen broccoli cuts, kale, leeks, red and green peppers, mustard greens, okra, onions, radishes, raw spinach (1/2 cup), summer squash, turnips, snow peas	Beet greens, cactus, cooked Chinese cabbage, Artichoke, fresh bamboo shoots, kohlrabi, rutabagas, tomatoes, tomato sauce or paste, sauerkraut , cooked spinach, tomato juice, vegetable juice

Higher-protein foods

Meats, cheeses and eggs

RECOMMENDED	AVOID
Lean cuts of meat, fish, poultry, and seafood; eggs, low cholesterol egg substitute; cottage cheese (limited due to high sodium content)	Bacon, cheeses, hot dogs, canned and luncheon meats, organ meats, salami, salmon, sausage, nuts, pepperoni

Higher-fat foods

Seasoning and calories

RECOMMENDED	AVOID
Tub or soft margarine low in trans fats, cream cheese, low fat mayonnaise, mayonnaise, sour cream, low fat cream cheese, low fat sour cream	Bacon fat, Crisco®, lard, shortening, back fat, butter, margarines high in trans fats, whipping cream

Beverages

RECOMMENDED	AVOID
Water, diet clear sodas, lemonade sweetened or homemade tea with an artificial sweetener	Regular or diet dark colas, fruit-flavored drinks or water sweetened with fruit juices, beer, fruit juices, bottled or lemonade containing sugar or or canned iced tea, syrup, or phosphoric acid; tea or lemonade sweetened with real sugar

You may also be instructed to avoid or limit the following salty and sweet foods:

- Honey
- Molasses
- Baked goods
- Candy
- Canned foods
- Condiments
- Onion, garlic or table salt
- Chocolate Regular sugar
- Syrup
- Ice cream
- TV dinners
- Meat tenderizer
- Salted chips and snacks
- Marinades
- Nuts
- Pizza

CONCLUSION

———— ⟋⟋ ————

A personalized nutrition program constitutes the basis of the treatment for diabetics to demonstrate a healthy and quality lifestyle. A good nutrition plan prepared especially for Type II diabetics is important for keeping blood sugar levels at normal levels.

Since every person is different from each other, the diets of individuals with diabetes require a difference according to their lifestyle. There is no single diet example for those with diabetes.

The most important point when preparing a diet plan should be to protect the body weight of the person with diabetes unless there is a contrary situation.

It should be fed at least 5 meals a day.

Protein, carbohydrates and fats should be included in the diet at levels that will meet the needs.

Alcohol consumption should be limited.

When the diet plan is prepared to be adequate and balanced, blood sugar remains at normal levels.

Some diabetics have been shown to improve their hypertension-related ailments by maintaining the correct body weights.

All the recipes in this book if used appropriately, will help make a good and balanced renal diet.

One that is low in phosphorus, protein, and sodium is a renal diet. The importance of eating high-quality protein and usually restricting fluids is often highlighted by a renal diet. The body of any person is different, so it is important for each patient to work with a renal dietitian to come up with a diet tailored to the needs of the patient.

To decrease the amount of waste in their blood, people with impaired kidney function must adhere to a renal or kidney diet. Blood waste comes from consumed food and liquids. The kidneys do not properly filter or remove waste when kidney function is impaired. When waste is left in the blood, it can adversely affect a patient's electrolyte levels. It can also help to boost kidney function and, by following a kidney diet, delay the onset of complete kidney failure.

CPSIA information can be obtained
at www.ICGtesting.com
Printed in the USA
BVHW010946021220
594591BV00022B/17

9 781801 256100